DR. BAHR'S
ACU-DIET

DR. BAHR'S ACU-DIET Weight Loss at Your Fingertips

THE 10-SECOND-A-DAY ACUPRESSURE REDUCING AND DIET BOOK

by Dr. Frank R. Bahr

TRANSLATED FROM THE GERMAN BY PAULA ARNO

WILLIAM MORROW AND COMPANY, INC.
NEW YORK   1978

Library of Congress Cataloging in Publication Data

Bahr, Frank R (date)
    Dr. Bahr's acu-diet.

    1. Reducing diets.   2. Acupressure.
I. Title.   II. Title: Acu-diet.
RM222.2.B3413   613.2′5   78-5949
ISBN 0-688-03307-5

BOOK DESIGN   CARL WEISS

Printed in the United States of America.

First Edition

1   2   3   4   5   6   7   8   9   10

PREFACE

It does not exactly further the prestige of a doctor engaged in scientific research when he writes a book that can be understood by everyone and is meant for everyone—in a word, a popular book about a medical subject. I do this because overweight has become *the* risk factor for the health of the individual, and this fact simply *has* to be driven home.

What matters is that all concerned realize the peril inherent in their excessive, unhealthful poundage, and the need for getting rid of it healthfully and lastingly. That is why I do not write in scientific jargon for a restricted circle of readers, but write the book in such a way that everyone can understand it and—equally important—can read it without getting bored. I hope that this is what the book will accomplish.

Dr. Frank R. Bahr
Munich, November 1977

CONTENTS

PREFACE   5

■ Overweight—Not Only a Question of Looks   11

■ Fat People Live Dangerously   11

◪ Ideal Weight, Overweight   13

■ We Eat Much Too Much—But Why?   15

■ The Man at the Control Panel Still Eats As His
Great-grandfather Ate   17

■ Stress Awakens the Appetite   18

■ But What Is Stress?   19

■ An Ill-advised Custom: The Banquet   20

■ The Control Mechanism Fails—Eating Becomes
an Addiction   21

■ It Can't Be Done Without a Diet, but Dieting Alone
Won't Do It   23

■ The Problem Is—the Habit Can't Be Broken   25

■ Acupressure—What Is That?   26

8 /

■ The Ten-Second Method, or, Have You Met Pavlov's
Dogs? 29

■ Pavlov's Experiment Turned Around: Conditioning
Against Compulsive Eating 29

■ Locating the Right Acupressure Points 30

■ The Direction of the Massage 31

■ The Pressure 31

■ Are You a Compulsive Eater? 31

■ The Overeater's Acupressure 32

■ Does Acupressure Suppress All Oral Reflexes? 36

■ The Overeater's Acupressure Stickers 37

■ While You Are Fasting, Do You Often Have a Strange
Hollow Feeling in Your Stomach Area? 37

■ Do You Eat to Compensate for Depression? 38

■ Do You Eat Mainly After Stress? 42

■ Do You Overeat for Other Reasons? 44

■ Acupressure: The Method for Everyone 45

■ Dangers from Excessive or Neurotic Use of Acupressure 47

■ And Now: The Diet 47

■ Crash Diets Are Not Necessary 51

■ Everything Slims You Down! 52

■ What Does the Body Need? What Can It Do Without? 55

■ Which Diet with Acupressure? 58

■ The Ideal Combination 58

■ Why Is the Combination of Protein and Raw Vegetables
So Important?   60

■ Keeping Your Bowels Functioning   61

■ Why Multivitamin Tablets Instead of Fruit During
the Starter Diet?   61

■ Necessary: Blood-Pressure Checks   62

■ Yes! You Made It! You Are Rid of the First Few
Pounds!   63

■ Beverages   64

■ The 800-Calorie Reducing Diet: Recipes   65

■ Reduced Enough? Desired Weight Achieved?   90

■ Beverages   92

■ The Weight-Maintenance Diet: Recipes   93

■ Acupressure—As the Patients See It   121

■ Exercise, Exercise, Exercise!   127

■ The Idle Wheel Rusts   128

■ What Are My Limits?   130

■ Exercises Aimed at Critical Points—Exercises That
You Will Enjoy!   137

■ Too Indolent for a Few Seconds of Acupressure? How
Would You Like to Try Wire, Knife, and Electricity? 149

APPENDIX /   The Scientific Basis of Acupressure   153

INDEX   157

OVERWEIGHT—NOT ONLY
A QUESTION OF LOOKS

This excerpt from a female patient's letter tells a common story: ". . . I would like to lose my fat, and I would be grateful if that could be accomplished soon because I am going on vacation in June and would like to look more attractive by then . . ."

This is a typical attitude; most fat people are bothered mainly by their appearance, and very understandably so, since the current ideal of beauty, at least in the Western world, calls for a slim, trim figure. This beauty ideal is a most sensible one from a medical point of view. Regrettably, excess pounds damage more than a person's looks.

FAT PEOPLE LIVE DANGEROUSLY

Those overweight by 10 percent or more face five dangers:

Danger #1: Their heart is overburdened. To sustain the excess bulk, it has to pump up to forty more quarts of blood per hour. This blood, moreover, is often too fatty, with too high a cholesterol level. The result is twice the danger of suffering a cardiac infarction for the overweight, compared with people of normal weight.

Danger #2: Fat and carbohydrate metabolism in the overweight is often impaired. The chance of falling prey to metabolic disorders is four times as great for an overweight person as for a normal individual. We are not dealing here with mild or harmless disorders, but with diabetes, for instance, which as a rule hits the obese harder and earlier in life than it does the person of normal weight.

Danger #3: The obese suffer three times as often as normal people from high blood pressure, which in turn, as we all know by now, can have many disagreeable consequences such as an inclination to headaches, a decrease in work capacity, and disturbance of sleep, as well as painful heart cramps (angina pectoris) and cardiac infarcts.

Danger #4: In conjunction with metabolic disorders, three times as many overweight individuals suffer from gallstones, an affliction which certainly cannot be taken lightly; not only are gallbladder cramps among the most disagreeable of pains, but they also carry with them the risk of an operation.

Danger #5: Since a sizable share of the excess poundage is often due to a generous consumption of beer, wine, and hard liquor, the obese are also in the front ranks of the liver-damaged. This damage begins with a fatty liver, a condition that is still curable, and ends with an atrophied liver (cirrhosis), which causes no pain, but kills.

Taken all together, this means a drastic reduction of life expectancy for the overweight. Admittedly, it seldom happens that someone literally eats himself to death, as was the case recently with a young Bavarian man from Dingolfingen who had achieved a live weight of 684 pounds by the time heart failure carried him off at the age of twenty.

We could assume that rock idol Elvis Presley also died because of his overweight, of a cardiac infarction at the age of forty-two. According to the coroner, Dr. Jerry Francisco, the autopsy revealed the presence of eight different drugs in Mr. Presley's body, but they had nothing to do with his death. For years, Elvis Presley had been suffering from heart disease, his blood pressure had been too high, and he had been enormously overweight.

But even without any extremes, in cases of routine overweight, so to speak, there is a measurable shortening of life. A fairly reliable estimate is that every two pounds of excess weight shortens the average life expectancy by four months. The by no means rare thirty pounds of excess fat cost, therefore, roughly five years of one's life.

This is a veritable catalogue of horrors, familiar, one would think, to all our overweight fellow citizens since almost every newspaper and popular magazine regularly points to the dangers of obesity and recommends various low-calorie recipes.

But, strangely enough, this does not help. The National Center for Health Statistics recently reported that American men and women in most age and height groups weigh more than they did fifteen years ago. They reported that 41.9 percent of women surveyed think they are at the ideal weight; 48.9 percent think they are overweight; 6.2 percent think they are underweight; 3.1 percent had no opinion. 51 percent of men think they are at the ideal weight; 30.5 percent think they are overweight; 9.6 percent think they are underweight; 8.9 percent had no opinion.

It is not at all exaggerated, therefore, to call overweight, or obesity, a dangerous epidemic. It truly is a plague that cries for relief.

IDEAL WEIGHT, OVERWEIGHT

A person's ideal weight is the weight at which he or she lives longest. This weight was determined a few years ago by a group of major life insurance companies. They ran hundreds of thousands of their insurance cases through a computer, discarded all those involving accidental deaths and deaths resulting from other external causes, and thus found out which of those covered lived longest. They were those who weighed 10 percent less than their so-called normal weight. Since then, a body weight of about 10 pounds less than normal has been designated as ideal weight. Thus, the ideal weight of a man five feet nine inches tall with a medium frame would be a little under 150 pounds.

But calculating the desirable weight only on the basis of height is too crude a method because human bones may vary considerably in thickness and weight. Moreover, one person has broader shoulders than the next, or a much narrower pelvis; ribs can be flat and short or very curved and correspondingly longer. At equal height, difference in bone structure can account for a weight difference of up to 20 pounds, especially in very tall people.

These factors are taken into account in the adjacent table. If you do not know whether to consider your bone structure light, medium, or heavy (appearances can be deceptive) you would do best to ask your doctor. Since constitutionally determined differences occur within these three groups, variations are allowed for in the table. A man with heavy bone structure, six feet one inch tall, weighing 168 pounds, actually does not need to read any further because he is at his ideal weight. But such cases are rare. Only 10 percent to, at most, 15 percent of all people are at their ideal weight.

DESIRABLE WEIGHTS FOR MEN AND WOMEN
According to Height and Frame, Ages 25 and Over

HEIGHT (in Shoes)*	Weight in Pounds (In Indoor Clothing)		
	SMALL FRAME	MEDIUM FRAME	LARGE FRAME
MEN			
5′ 2″	112-120	118-129	126-141
3″	115-123	121-133	129-144
4″	118-126	124-136	132-148
5″	121-129	127-139	135-152
6″	124-133	130-143	138-156
7″	128-137	134-147	142-161
8″	132-141	138-152	147-166
9″	136-145	142-156	151-170
10″	140-150	146-160	155-174
11″	144-154	150-165	159-179
6′ 0″	148-158	154-170	164-184
1″	152-162	158-175	168-189
2″	156-167	162-180	173-194
3″	160-171	167-185	178-199
4″	164-175	172-190	182-204

HEIGHT (in Shoes)*	Weight in Pounds (In Indoor Clothing)		
	SMALL FRAME	MEDIUM FRAME	LARGE FRAME
WOMEN			
4' 10"	92- 98	96-107	104-119
11"	94-101	98-110	106-122
5' 0"	96-104	101-113	109-125
1"	99-107	104-116	112-128
2"	102-110	107-119	115-131
3"	105-113	110-122	118-134
4"	108-116	113-126	121-138
5"	111-119	116-130	125-142
6"	114-123	120-135	129-146
7"	118-127	124-139	133-150
8"	122-131	128-143	137-154
9"	126-135	132-147	141-158
10"	130-140	136-151	145-163
11"	134-144	140-155	149-168
6' 0"	138-148	144-159	153-173

* 1-inch heels for men and 2-inch heels for women.

Note: Prepared by the Metropolitan Life Insurance Company. Derived primarily from data of the *Build and Blood Pressure Study, 1959*, Society of Actuaries.

WE EAT MUCH TOO MUCH—BUT WHY?

The cause of widespread and health-endangering overweight is as simple as can be: Whoever hits the scale at too many pounds eats too much—and probably the wrong food as well—and/or drinks too much alcohol.

That's all there is to it.

The favorite explanation of the overweight, which they try so hard to believe themselves—that the bulging fat they carry around their middle is the result of some glandular dysfunction or of an allergy—simply doesn't work any longer. Painstaking studies have shown that instances where obesity is due to a purely physiological dysfunction are rare indeed. They do not even account for 1 percent of all cases of overweight.

Why, then, do so many people inflict this damage upon

themselves and others? (Every fourth child is overfed.) There are many and intricate reasons for this; some lie in the remotest past, others in the more recent past, and quite a few in the present.

From our primeval past stems our ability to store energy reserves in the form of fat in our own bodies, an ability which we have in common with almost all animal species, be they mammals, birds, or fish.

For our earliest ancestors this capacity was super-vital; they were hunters who stalked monsters like the mighty mammoth or the powerful bison, and when they had brought one down, they stored the nutritional value in their own bodies, for the refrigerator had not yet been invented. So they ate for days and rejoiced in their body fat. They certainly needed it; it could be a long time between mammoths.

In those days, our double system of utilizing nutrition made eminently good sense: Man can take from outside his body the energy which he constantly needs to maintain the correct body temperature, to keep up his various bodily functions, to move and to work—by eating. But when there is no energy available from outside, he can nourish himself from within, by breaking down stored fats, and in extreme cases even muscles and connective tissue. Before a man starves to death, he first consumes a part of himself.

Although the atavistic, programmed storage economy of our organism, which causes it to hoard even the slightest excess energy as fat, is bothersome today, it nevertheless has its advantages. Without the capacity for internal nourishment, it would be even harder than it already is to get rid of the piled-on overweight.

But something else has been passed on to us from our ancestors: the lust for eating. For hairy proto-man, who seldom had enough to eat, every meal must have been a mighty feast, since nature has purposefully coupled all important functions that preserve the species and the individual with pleasure feelings—and the more essential the function, the more intense the pleasure. Reproduction and eating are the most important of these functions and therefore are also the most lustful pursuits.

THE MAN AT THE CONTROL PANEL STILL EATS AS HIS GREAT-GRANDFATHER ATE

A good part of our eating habits are an inheritance from a far less distant past. In this context, the word "inheritance" should not be taken too literally, since habits, strictly speaking, cannot be inherited. But they are transmitted from generation to generation with about the same consistency as true hereditary material. If one asks young women today how they cook, the answer in ninety out of a hundred cases will be "like my mother."

Today's woman relies heavily on canned or frozen foods, whereas her mother made her own spaghetti sauce and baked homemade pies. But these differences are only technical, not qualitative—and if one had asked the mother and grandmother of today's woman where their cooking methods came from, the answer would have been the same. Not only do "laws and rights multiply like an evil disease," as Goethe wrote—so also do eating habits.

Until a few generations ago, most people spent their lives in hard physical labor. Masons lugged stones and cement up scaffoldings on their backs; there was no crane to do it for them. Miners hacked coal from the face of mine galleries. Cow barns were mucked out by pitchfork, not conveyor belt, and in the fields the farmer did not sit in the comfortable cab of a 150-horsepower tractor, but walked behind the plow, and although this was pulled by a team of horses or oxen, he had to press it into the furrow with considerable effort and force it to move in a straight line. It is easy to imagine what a sweaty occupation that was!

All this hard labor called for appropriate nourishment—indeed, for a lot of food and fat, at that. At such a high energy-consumption level, this did no harm; on the contrary, under these circumstances fatty bacon was a welcome energy food. But times have changed. Today, the number of those who must still perform true heavy labor has fallen to a minimum. The great-grandchildren of those former toilers now stand in white smocks before control panels or even sit in front of them. But unchanged are the eating habits, the far too energy-rich heavy diet.

To illustrate, here are a few figures: The average energy requirement for men today is about 2,500 calories, for women about 2,200 calories. But men usually eat the equivalent of about 3,100 calories, women about 2,610. Since these average figures comprise those who eat sensibly or even less, the average daily consumption of the overweight members of the population must be more like 3,600 calories for men and 3,000 calories for women, or almost 40 percent too high. Small wonder that heavy rolls of fat decorate so many hips.

The average consumption of fat also lies far above the necessary level: men, on the average, eat five and a half ounces of fat per day and women four ounces. Under a normal work load, two and a half to three ounces would be quite sufficient for both men and women. Two ounces of fat per day too many add up to almost four pounds of overweight a month.

STRESS AWAKENS THE APPETITE

To the prehistoric factors that seduce so many into overeating must be added a few contemporary ones. It begins with the newborn. Baby cries. Perhaps it is hungry. Perhaps it just wants tenderness, some attention. But it gets a bottle every time—breast feeding hardly exists anymore. And look at that—baby drinks and is contented. Truly? Can milk, or more precisely, can a high-grade baby formula, substitute for love?

NO. But the baby gets used to it and demands food when it is in need of love. Substitute gratification is the name for this. And this tendency remains with the baby when it has long ceased to be one, but has become an adult. Anger, tension, frustration—she or he makes straight for the cooky jar, the candy box, the beer can. This is what is commonly called "nervous eating." The result is a sort of "grievance fat."

To top all this off, there is the notorious stress that besets us all, the pupil as well as the teacher, the workman at the assembly line as much as the manager harassed by telephones and deadlines, the patient in the overcrowded waiting room as well as the doctor next door.

BUT WHAT IS STRESS?

The ability to react unerringly to stress was a dire necessity for a Stone Age man, forced to escape from a wild beast that suddenly came upon him. It is also stress reaction when a feeble pencil-pusher avoids an onrushing car by a mighty leap, a feat that he could otherwise never accomplish.

Stress reaction within the body's warning system is programmed for maximum effort. This always works, in all humans, along the following lines. The brain receives threatening information via the sense organs and, via nerve pathways, orders the suprarenal medulla to pour adrenalin into the bloodstream. Thereby, blood pressure and rate of heartbeat are raised with lightning speed to insure the increased oxygen supply needed to produce the energy for a fight-or-flight reaction. In contrast, digestion is switched off, since it would only waste energy in a moment of danger. In split seconds enormous energy resources are freed, enabling man to make maximum efforts that he would not be capable of under norman conditions, but that save his life in danger, in battle, or during a conflagration.

It is a pity that today these stress reactions are triggered by all sorts of not really threatening irritants like trouble at the office, a fight with one's spouse, a rattling pneumatic hammer outside one's door, a traffic accident. To an already irritated mind, even a train delay is enough to release a stress reaction.

The trouble is that the organism gets into a state of alarm and tension that cannot be reduced in the manner we are provided with—who would, after all, hoist his desk in the air after a reprimand from the boss, or run full speed ten times around the block after a clash with her mother-in-law? It would be beneficial; it would work off the tension; but it is rarely feasible. That leaves those who are plagued by stress to work it off in other ways. And very many people do so by choosing to eat something.

It is entirely possible that this compulsory eating after stress is still part of the stress reaction: The organism believes —erroneously—that it has to replace the readied great energy, when, in fact, it has not used it up. Be that as it may, with many people stress is certainly the reason for their eating more than is good for them.

AN ILL-ADVISED CUSTOM: THE BANQUET

The habit of celebrating anything and everything—birthday, promotion, club anniversary—with a banquet also contributes to the intake of too many calories. Such a feast is usually abundant; alcoholic beverages are rarely missing, and it frequently takes place in the evening. This is a time when the body, because it will soon rest for a prolonged period, uses hardly any energy and transforms the ingested calories into stored fat at an especially high rate. Activities like dancing after a rich evening meal can hardly make up for this fact.

There are more than enough reasons for overeating. But are they really so compelling that half of the population cannot resist them? Or are there still other contributing factors?

THE CONTROL MECHANISM FAILS—
EATING BECOMES AN ADDICTION

Actually it is hard to understand. The human organism is an all-but-incredible miracle of the finest and most perfect regulatory mechanisms. It can accurately maintain its ideal operating temperature to a tenth of a degree in cold and hot weather; it adjusts respiratory rate and heart rhythm precisely to the requirements; it can safely govern the most complicated sequels of motion; and the speed of its reflexes lies in the supersonic range—to give just a few examples. What happens in the more minute hormonal and nerve regions is far more intricate and complicated, but always calibrated to a degree that all the computers in the world could not match.

Should not such a marvel be able to regulate its own energy replenishment precisely according to need, taking in not a calorie too many, not one too few? Well, we do have the suitable control mechanism. It is located in the midbrain above the terminus of the extended spinal cord and deep inside the skull. This whole region of the brain is, on the one hand, the gateway for our consciousness: All sensory perceptions pass through here, are "processed" and tagged with sensations of pleasure or pain, and then are passed on to the corresponding area of the cerebrum. On the other hand, its lower part (hypothalamus) is also the most important control center for all autonomous processes like breathing, heartbeat, temperature regulation, sleep and waking rhythm, and the like. Expressed differently, the hypothalamus is the steering center of the autonomic nervous system.

Our attitude toward eating, the feeling of hunger or satiety, is controlled in this region. True hunger—not appetite—cannot be brought about voluntarily; one is hungry or isn't depending on what is being signaled from the hypothalamus. In animal experiments, it is possible to pinpoint precisely where in the hypothalamus the feeding centers are located:

If one stimulates a certain spot (through electricity or injections), the test animals start to eat without restraint and get fatter as you watch. Stimulation of another specific point causes the animals to refuse all food and, without countermeasures, they would simply starve to death.

A fully functioning control mechanism does, indeed, exist, but in many people it obviously doesn't work as it should. The right control would mean that hunger and appetite would lead to food intake only when the first signs of deficiency, lowering of the blood-sugar level, for instance, made this seem advisable; and, furthermore, that all additional food intake would be prevented by a feeling of satiety or disgust.

Everyone knows that it doesn't happen that way—the control mechanism fails. To be more precise, it *seems* to fail. It would be better to say that the control of our eating habits is not geared to present-day conditions. The parts of our brain that are in charge of this control are among the oldest in our evolutionary history; there are many indications that they are programmed to function in a situation of constant scarcity— just those circumstances in which early man, living in a hunting society, always found himself.

This brings us to what we call appetite: the desire to eat when one is not actually hungry. Not real hunger, but the mere sight of something edible triggers one's appetite. Be it only an illustration in one of the many richly colored magazines on the art of cooking, it causes one's "mouth to water" and the gastric juices to flow; the body immediately readies itself for food intake.

This is a fatal scenario in a situation where food is continuously and plentifully available. Its effect can be clearly seen in domestic animals. In the brain of a dog or a cat there exists that same "eat-when-you-can-so-you-won't-want-later" program. As long as animals live in the wilds and have to hunt their own food, this works perfectly; no wild animal will ever get fat unless it is getting ready for hibernation. But as soon as a dog or a cat becomes domesticated and has a continuous food supply, it eats—if permitted to do so—without restraint, and immediately becomes fat, with the same dire consequences as in humans, including cardiac infarction.

But what does this failure of the controls mean? It means that overeating can become compulsive, that the "feeding center" of the brain under these changed conditions has become a "food-addiction center," and that hazardous overeating has turned into addiction.

This does not mean that all people are equally affected in this manner. The lucky ones who always stay at their normal or ideal weight have retained a well-functioning regulator in their feeding center, with a food intake governed by hunger and not by appetite. Normally, this feeding center in the brain works perfectly in children who have not been forced by their mothers always to clean their plates; as soon as the feeling of hunger is gone, the child stops eating. Such children are not overweight. The fault lies, therefore, mostly with the mothers who, thinking "my child must have the best," are doing precisely the wrong thing.

This book is for those who want to fight their overweight, those who—often despairingly—struggle against their urge to eat, without ever achieving more than a temporary result. They are true addicts, and only if they are treated as such, and also see themselves as such, can they be helped.

IT CAN'T BE DONE WITHOUT A DIET, BUT DIETING ALONE WON'T DO IT

It is obvious to anyone: Whoever has piled on one or two dozen pounds of overweight can only lose them again by means of a low-calorie diet. It may be possible also to work off the pounds by strenuous exercise, but this would require so great an effort even in the case of comparatively minor overweight (compare table on page 14) that reducing solely in this way is not practicable.

After all, there are sensible diets. The relevant literature fills whole libraries; diet suggestions and methods number in the hundreds. In most instances they even carry guarantees. One example:

Of all the patients who stayed with the diet program and the instructions connected with it, as suggested by Dr. X, 80 percent had maintained the aimed-for weight after one year.

Such statements require careful scrutiny. "Of all . . . those who stayed with the program. . . ." How many were they? What percentage of those who started one or the other of the diet regimens have stuck with it in the long run? The diet books won't tell, and with good reason: The number is disturbingly small.

When weight is lost through dieting without let-up, great is the joy when the desired weight has been achieved, bitter the disappointment when after a while the indicator on the scale slowly climbs again to higher figures and finally reaches the old position. According to a recent study that evaluated 20,000 cases, this is the sad truth in 95 percent of all cases where overweight people have, at first successfully, reduced by means of a diet.

The number of overweight people does not go down, but up. That can only mean that hundreds of thousands have had the depressing experience of having been able to reduce, but unable to maintain a healthy weight. The resulting disappointment, the feeling of being inferior because of lack of willpower, drives many to start filling their plates with a vengeance.

Not everyone accepts the situation as calmly as one of my patients who, with cheerful laughter, summed up his experiences as follows: "If I add up all the pounds I have lost in the last few years, there really isn't anything left of me." What was left, though, was excess weight, living proof that by dieting one can, indeed, lose many pounds, but not the addiction. That remains, and causes the pounds to accumulate once more.

That is why diet alone cannot do the job. Only if one breaks down the fat with a balanced diet and *at the same time* treats the urge to overeat as an addiction and attacks it with my method can lasting success be expected.

THE PROBLEM IS—THE HABIT CAN'T BE BROKEN

Compulsive eating differs in one very important respect from other addictions—the habit can't be broken. Even a heavy smoker can give up smoking if he makes up his mind, really stops, and has enough willpower to stick to it. The first weeks may be rough, the following ones not much better, but eventually, little by little, the addiction becomes weaker—dries up, so to speak—until at last it disappears and the smoker is a smoker no longer. An alcoholic can also get rid of his habit. It doesn't happen very often; the high relapse percentage is only too well known. But, at least, it is possible. If an alcoholic is deprived of all liquor for a sufficiently long time, he too can be cured. At least theoretically, this holds true even for narcotics addicts; after a long abstinence, lasting perhaps several years (if that can be achieved), their addiction, too, will fade away. These habits can be broken, if the object of craving is strictly withheld from the addict.

Compulsive eating cannot be stopped that way. No one needs to smoke, tipple, or shoot heroin, but everyone has to eat. It isn't possible to separate the compulsive eater from the object of his craving. He would starve. For this reason compulsive eating can be treated only by attacking it "head on" at its starting point in the midbrain. There originate the superabundant impulses to eat. They have to be blocked; once they have been stopped, the excessive appetite is gone—and gone with it is the addiction.

The method by which everyone can easily achieve this is acupressure. My own method for sustained and permanent weight reduction is the combination *acupressure* plus *diet*.

ACUPRESSURE—WHAT IS THAT?

To begin with, a somewhat misleading word. It is a variation of the well-known concept "acupuncture"—the name, of Latin origin, for the ancient Chinese art of healing by needle pricks. In Latin *acus* means "needle," *punctum* "point," as well as "to prick," and *pressus* means "pressure"; *acupressure,* translated literally, means "needle pressure." Factually this is not correct, because needles are not involved. It should be named more appropriately "point pressure," "point pressing" or "point massage," since those terms describe the technique perfectly.

Yet, the name "acupressure" has become accepted, perhaps to stress the connection with acupuncture, since both procedures use the same points.

"Acupressure" is the name, then, for a method of soothing and healing pain and sickness through massage of certain indicated points on the body. This method is even older than acupuncture, which had its beginnings, as legend has it, under the reign of the Chinese emperor Huang Ti about 5,000 years ago. The body surface was pierced at points where, it had long been known—probably through chance discovery—the application of pressure would cause definite reactions inside the body.

The first written records of acupressure are of far more recent date. They can be found in a medical treatise from the time of the Chin Dynasty around the year 300 B.C. Certain stone utensils for massaging and tapping body points are described there; the Chinese name for them, *zehn-shi,* can be roughly translated as "stone needles." They probably were made of easily split stone, ground into pencil-shaped objects with rounded ends. At the time those records were made, acupuncture in China had already developed into an extensive system with hundreds of precisely defined points, along so-called body meridians, which were pierced with golden or silver needles, depending on the aimed-for result.

Western medicine long regarded Chinese acupuncture, of which it had not become aware until the seventeenth century, as a strange, dubious hocus-pocus. This rejection ended only recently, after it turned out that acupuncture's odd, point-laden "meridians" apparently correspond to functional connections in the cerebral cortex, that the Yin-Yang principle—you are healthy only as long as Yin (dark and weak) and Yang (light and strong) are in balance—could be a flowery circumlocution for the autonomic nervous system and its paired subsystems—the sympathetic and the parasympathetic—whose antithetic functions have to be in balance if the human organism is to function properly.

A short time ago it even became possible to objectively and scientifically identify the acupuncture points; they vary from their surrounding area by the skin's noticeably different electrical resistance and are usually perceptibly more sensitive to pressure than the adjacent skin.

Once the points were established with certainty, it was possible to prove the effects of acupuncture in animal tests. This method disproved the initial objections that acupuncture works only as long as one believes in it, or through autosuggestion. An animal can't fancy that it has no pains just because a vet stuck a few needles into its hide. Even Caesarean sections on beef cattle have been performed solely under acupuncture anesthesia by a veterinarian in Austria. In the United States there are several acupuncture veterinary hospitals used primarily for the treatment of valuable racehorses.

Acupuncture is being used more and more in private medical practice and at university hospitals. The practitioner must, of course, be thoroughly trained in this method. In Germany, some 3,000 major operations have been performed successfully under acupuncture anesthesia, mainly on patients who were unable to undergo the traditional methods of anesthesia.

How acupuncture works has been explained to a large extent through the cooperation of researchers in various fields of the sciences in the United States, Canada, China, Germany and

Austria. Briefly summarized: Free nerve endings are located under the skin at the acupuncture points. Stimulation of these points by needle pricks releases impulses that travel via the respective nerve pathways and the spine into the brain stem and on to the midbrain. There, in a netlike brain structure and in the nonspecific nuclei of the midbrain, the impulses are processed and release corresponding effects through neurophysiological reflexes and neurochemical substances that serve as transmitters of information.

Acupressure's effects and mode of action are in principle the same as in acupuncture. The only, and for us essential difference, is that the results achieved with needles are very strong, at times dramatic. For this reason, only a fully trained physician should be entrusted with the acupuncture needle. It is not enough, for example, to only free from excruciating pain, through acupuncture, a man with severe disc trouble whose vertebrae are already deformed. Such a patient has to be thoroughly apprised of the fact that he cannot kick up his heels now as if his spine were completely intact. Were he to do so, he would risk a slipped disk and, with it, agonizing nerve pressure. In extreme cases even paraplegia could develop. Similarly, no responsible doctor would try to eliminate pains in the abdominal region with acupuncture without having fully reassured himself that he is not dealing with an inflamed appendix or Fallopian tube, when only an operation would be the correct therapy.

These two examples, to which any number of others could be added, should suffice to make it clear that the acupuncture needle is not an instrument that can be handed to just anyone to play around with indiscriminately.

The situation is different in the case of acupressure. The fingertip pressure exerted here only massages a point on the body, and could never injure organs situated close to the subcutaneous tissue. Self-administration for certain purposes is, therefore, harmless. Especially beneficial is the use of acupressure for the curbing of the compulsive-eating center. One can, of course, go after the urge to eat with acupuncture, and shackle it very effectively, but this is only necessary in extreme and exceptional cases.

Such patients may turn to the German Academy for Auricular Medicine, U.S.A., 3904 Boonson Boulevard, Kalamazoo, Michigan, 49008, for a list of acupuncture physicians (enclose stamped, self-addressed envelope).

THE TEN-SECOND METHOD, OR, HAVE YOU MET PAVLOV'S DOGS?

"Pavlov, Ivan Petrovich, Russian medical scientist . . . 1904 Nobel Prize for Medicine . . . died 1936 . . . discovered the *conditioned reflexes* and how to train them. . . ."

On the title page of our book it says: "The Ten-Second-a-Day Acupressure Reducing and Diet Book." This bold announcement that ten-second-a-day acupressure massages can effectively restrain the compulsive-eating center has a lot to do with the old Grand Master Pavlov. Let's recall what Professor Pavlov found out. He fed dogs—and very well, too. The dogs started to salivate at the mere sight of their tasty meal. At the same time, Pavlov let a bell ring in a certain key. Eventually, Professor Pavlov had only to ring the bell and his dogs would begin to salivate without any food in sight. Proof of the conditioned reflex, of the capacity to habituate responses, had been established. Conditioning takes time, but works dependably.

PAVLOV'S EXPERIMENT TURNED AROUND: CONDITIONING AGAINST COMPULSIVE EATING

In the overeater's acupressure, the increasing conditioning results in reinforcement of the acupressure effect and finally in a drastic reduction of the necessary acupressure effort. In practice it looks this way: The overweight person who begins to curb his urge to eat by point massage—you'll find out in detail in the next chapter how this is done—will at first need quite some time until he checks the very lively activity of his compulsive-eating center enough to notice any effect and to feel his appetite disappear. That may take longer than the indicated ten seconds, at first; in extreme cases it could take considerably longer.

But happily, the required time steadily decreases at the same rate as the reflex paths leading from the massaged points to the midbrain become well established. The effect of the acupressure, not very noticeable during the first days of treatment, will also become increasingly stronger. After one week, only half the time required at the beginning will be necessary; after another week, the time needed is halved again, and so forth. Progressive conditioning leads to a point where ten seconds of acupressure are enough to thoroughly kill the appetite.

It is indispensable, though, that one use acupressure *every day*, otherwise the reflex paths will not become conditioned in the manner described earlier.

LOCATING THE RIGHT ACUPRESSURE POINTS

In principle, points that release the described reflexes in the brain are massaged. When you practice acupressure, it is of the utmost importance to correctly locate the points. The more exact you are in massaging precisely the right point, the stronger will be the effect. When first leafing through the book, you may have noticed that several photographs help to clarify the text, and they will make it easy for you to locate the points. For the best possible acupressure results, please always simultaneously use all three methods for locating a point.

Method #1: Look very carefully at the photographs and find the point or points on your own body (visual identification).

Method #2: Read, word for word, the related text in which the manner of locating the point is described and, following the instructions in the text, find the corresponding acupressure point (combined visual and manual identification).

Method #3: To be absolutely sure of finding the right acupressure point make use of the fact that the spot to be located is more sensitive to pressure than its surrounding area. Determined pressure with a finger will be felt more strongly at the acupressure point than in its vicinity (pressure-sensitive identification).

THE DIRECTION OF THE MASSAGE

Once you have found the point, you have to massage it in the indicated direction, not just rub back and forth on the skin. The Chinese, with their thousands of years of experience with acupressure, warn that acupressure in the wrong direction is senseless. The explanation for this is plain. The acupressure points are situated along directional energy routes, the so-called meridians. These clearly determine the necessary direction. The photos and the text in this book carefully indicate the correct direction.

THE PRESSURE

Keep in mind that you want to release a reflex; to achieve this, the free nerve endings in the skin have to be stimulated. This means the pressure definitely has to be felt, but you do not want to injure your skin or massage yourself black and blue. Sufficient pressure is important, especially during the first days of acupressure treatment. Later on you may progressively reduce the pressure, making sure it remains perceptible, since the effect of conditioning, once the reflex paths have become habituated, reinforces the effect of the massage.

ARE YOU A COMPULSIVE EATER?

Most fat people are. One patient told me before her treatment that she once was so irresistibly overcome by her craving that she begged a total stranger in a restaurant for a bite of his fragrant pork roast because she did not have enough money with her for a meal, having entered the restaurant only for a quick cup of coffee.

How can you tell that you are a compulsive eater? Check your answer to the following questions:

yes no Can you pass by a store with a window display of tempting goodies? Or are you driven to enter the store and buy something, although what drives you is not hunger, just appetite?

yes no Do you ask yourself after a substantial lunch or dinner, What else would taste good now?—Perhaps an ice cream or a candy bar?

yes no Do you feel propelled toward the refrigerator, although you are not the least bit hungry, when you are watching someone on TV happily stuffing himself?

yes no Does the mere sight of a full-color photo of a gourmet dish make you ravenously hungry?

If you have answered more than one of the questions with "yes," then acupressure makes sense for you and will serve your purpose.

THE OVEREATER'S ACUPRESSURE

You will notice in the photo, that the acupressure point is located exactly midway between nose and upper lip—but this point is not on the outside of the upper lip, it is on the inside. As seen from the interior of the mouth, it is about one four-hundredth of an inch under the mucous membrane of the upper lip (see schematic drawing).

The point is well hidden, indeed. That is why the Chinese never discovered it and could not include it in their acupuncture charts. I found this point only by chance, while systematically investigating the whole mouth area of one of my patients. This point becomes amazingly effective only after the reflex pathways to the brain have become conditioned by acupressure for two or three days. To massage it, you have to use a little trick.

Since the point is hidden on the inside of the upper lip, one

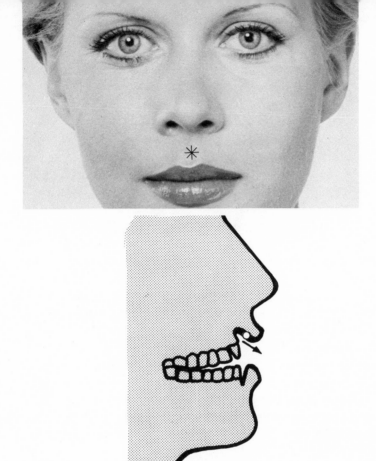

could, of course, use the thumb and the tip of the middle finger in a pincer-like movement, with the thumb inside the lip, the middle finger outside. To massage, the thumb would move a little downward (about an eighth of an inch) while the middle finger would move slightly upward. The point acting upon the compulsion is then actually inside the pincers formed by the fingers, and is being massaged in a downward motion on the inside of the lip while the outside of the lip moves upward. When you are in the bathtub in the morning, and have just cleaned your teeth and thoroughly washed your hands, then why don't you try pincer acupressure. This point, however, only

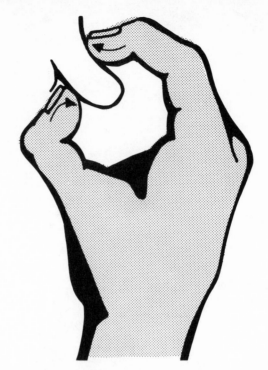

becomes so unbelievably effective after two or three days, at which time the reflex passages to the brain have become programmed.

PINCER ACUPRESSURE

Since the acupressure on the upper lip is hidden on the inside, you could, of course, pull the lip slightly forward with the left hand and then massage the point on the inside with the index finger of the right hand. An alternative to this is to use the pincer acupressure technique.

This technique utilizes the thumb and index finger in a vise-like fashion: The thumb is inside the lip and the index finger is outside. You then massage so that the thumb is somewhat below the index finger (about a fraction of an inch) which is then rotated. The compulsion point should then be located between the thumb and the index finger, which together form a vise. It is this viselike action which causes the effects of the massage to be so immediate and powerful. The point is actually massaged on the inside of the lip from top to bottom. At the same time the outside of the lip is massaged conversely from bottom to top. After you have brushed your teeth in the morning and your hands are clean, you should follow through with this pincer acupressure routine every day.

True, you don't spend your days standing with freshly scrubbed hands in the bathtub. You go to work, and it would not be hygienic to reach into your mouth with hands that have just operated a photocopier or a typewriter. So, here is the little trick:

With the nail of your index finger you press, on the outside, the midpoint between nose and upper lip. You may dimly remember that you were told in school, during physics class, that pressure equals counterpressure. That is correct. When you now slowly exert pressure, you feel the counterpressure on the inside of the lip where it rests on the upper jaw.

When you now move *the whole upper lip* with the nail of your index finger upward by about an eighth of an inch, without changing the main point on which the nail of your index finger rests, but while exerting pressure, then you will feel how our acupressure point on the inside of the lip is being beautifully massaged by the counterpressure of the upper jaw.

With your index finger you carry out this small, fast, upward shifting of the lip (about thirty movements or more) for ten seconds, or perhaps a little longer at first. The point itself, on the inside of the lip, will then be massaged downward, just as it was massaged by the thumb in the pincer acupressure. This sounds much more complicated than it really is; why don't you just give it a quick try.

Here is a little acupressure trick for today. Here you are on the assembly line in Detroit, or maybe you have dirty hands for some other reason, when the urge to eat hits you. You search for an alternative.

Nothing easier. You take a pencil or ballpoint pen and press on the described point, using the rounded end. Again, be careful not to slip on the outside of the lip while moving, with pressure, *the whole lip* upward by about an eighth of an inch. The acupressure point on the inside will be massaged splendidly by counterpressure from the upper jaw.

While you are using the rounded end of a pencil as a substitute for your fingertip, you also make thirty upward motions in about ten seconds. At the beginning, and until the reflexes are well conditioned, you acupress, if need be, a little longer. The movement is not unlike the pecking of a bird, but the direction is not straight at the teeth, but obliquely upward.

For ten seconds, then (perhaps a little longer in the beginning), quickly repeat these small lip manipulations toward the top (approximately thirty movements or more). Thus the point, located on the inside of the lip, will be almost as effectively massaged as it is in the pincer technique with the thumb. This sounds like it's more complicated than it actually is, so why don't you just try it now.

As you can see, you can practice the overeater's acupressure *inconspicuously* even in your office or at any kind of work. Who doesn't once in a while play distractedly with a pencil? But once you have reached your ideal weight, be fair, and share our method with your co-workers. Be sure, though, to point out that acupressure only curbs compulsive eating; a low-calorie diet is the other, equally important factor in reducing.

DOES ACUPRESSURE SUPPRESS ALL ORAL REFLEXES?

No, the pleasure of kissing, for example, remains intact. The control point for that is nowhere near, but is located in the little valley between lower lip and chin, right in the center. If you want a little more excitement on that score, there is the spot to massage with an upward motion. Nor does anti-overeating acupressure impair any other sexual functions. Far from it: When the fat goes, a deterrent goes.

THE OVEREATER'S ACUPRESSURE STICKERS

I am sure, my patients are sure, and soon you too will be sure that the ideal method for slimming down is, without a doubt, my overeater's acupressure.

Of course, you'll have to devote to it the few seconds necessary. To turn the intention into the deed, you had better paste the enclosed stickers in the following places right now:

a) on the refrigerator door, as reliable help against weakening resolve;
b) even on the kitchen door;
c) on or next to a full-length mirror where you can see yourself from head to toe;
d) on your desk drawer at your place of work, for instance, where you are accustomed to hiding your cookies.

The slogan on the sticker—"Eat less—acupress"—should inspire you to carry out the overeater's acupressure before every meal and whenever your resolve weakens.

WHILE YOU ARE FASTING, DO YOU OFTEN HAVE A STRANGE HOLLOW FEELING IN YOUR STOMACH AREA?

Small nerve endings in the stomach walls tell the brain how full the stomach is. They are called stretch receptors. They are also subject to conditioning. In the obese, they are practically always overstretched, which means that a glutton keeps on eating cheerfully although the stomach nerves have long ago begun signalling "enough."

A twenty-eight-year-old patient of mine, five feet eight inches tall, weighing 177 pounds, said to me recently: "I can put away incredible quantities of food and gain up to nine pounds over a weekend. But I never get sick to my stomach!" There must have been quite some stretch in the nerve receptors

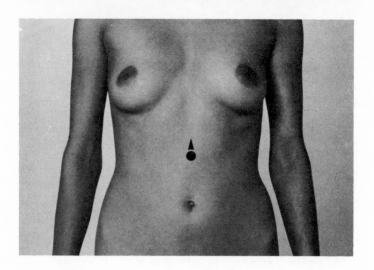

of this patient! She kept on eating merrily long after others had started to feel sick.

But the human organism is a wonderfully adaptable machine. If you begin to eat less, the stomach receptors will become adjusted and only during the transition period will you at times experience that strange hollow feeling in the stomach area.

To alleviate this condition, you can use a very simple acupressure point. You know where your navel is; now you can find it by touching your breastbone at its lower end. (This is easy even with a lot of fat covering your bones.) The acupressure point itself lies exactly halfway between your navel and the end of your breastbone (see photo). It has to be massaged upward. About thirty movements in ten seconds are normally amply sufficient. As a rule one massages the skin with the thumbnail in small, approximately inch-long strokes.

Pressure should be such that the skin is reddened after thirty massage strokes but the skin surface is not injured. This acupressure is to be employed after the overeater's acupressure on the upper lip, depending on need, three times a day or more.

DO YOU EAT TO COMPENSATE FOR DEPRESSION?

More and more people are seized by dejection and despondency. It is estimated that 30 percent of all illness is due to a depression syndrome. Regrettably, it is difficult to recognize the onset of depression since most of us, at one time or another, are discouraged and in low spirits, and since such spells in most cases go away by themselves. The disturbing aspect is that depression often hides behind other symptoms and becomes masked by an exaggerated urge to eat.

There are two main types of depression: the inherited, so-called endogenous depressions (in their case little can be expected from acupressure) and the self-induced (exogenous) depressions. Deviations of the brain's metabolism have been detected in the brain of depressives; these are now considered the main cause of depression.

Check the following:

yes	no	I frequently cry.
yes	no	I am often discouraged.
yes	no	I feel so lonely.
yes	no	I am often dejected.
yes	no	My life makes no sense.
yes	no	I have at times considered taking my own life.

If you have said "yes" to any of the above, you should, without fail, see a doctor. He will most likely prescribe antidepressant drugs.

But you know, of course, that drugs have side effects. You should, therefore, use acupressure against depression, after consultation with your doctor, to reduce drug intake to a minimum. The following acupressure is used *after* the over-eater's acupressure massage on the upper lip. As a general rule you have to massage the points on both the left and right sides of your body. The main pressure point used is the one that stimulates heart and psyche—called in Chinese *shao-chong* ("turbulence center of a wave")—close to the root of the nail, on the ring-finger side of the little finger; massage it across the finger toward the outside. The second main point is the *tung-li* ("connection with the inner life"), one and a

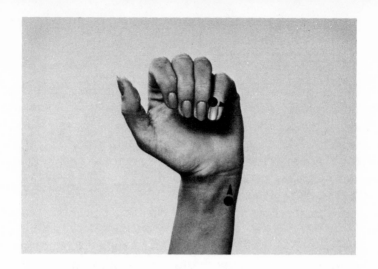

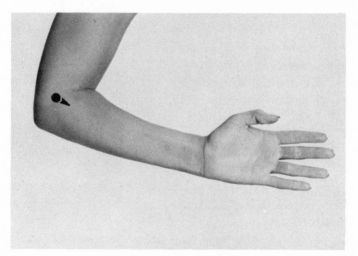

half to two finger widths above the wrist. Acupress it in the direction of the inside of the little finger.

The next point is known by its Chinese name, *shao-hai* ("small dewy sea of energy"). It also goes under the beautiful and appropriate epithet "point of vivaciousness." We chose this point for our front cover illustration for just this reason: Your vivaciousness will return after you have lost your first few pounds by using my method!

The "point of vivaciousness" is found on the inner end of the elbow fold, which is formed when your elbow is com-

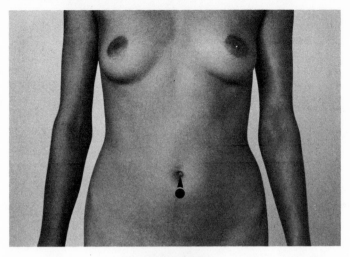

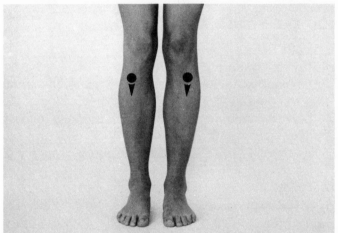

pletely bent. The point must be acupressed in the direction of the hand. This point is especially indicated when you are completely devoid of energy; it's for this reason that athletes secretly use this point in order to achieve optimal performance. The point has the added advantage of being an appetite depressant.

During periods characterized by a severe lack of vitality, the main point of energy, *ch'i-hai*, is recommended. It lies two to three finger widths below the navel. Massage it upward.

In case of restlessness during depression, make use of the point *tsu-san-li* ("Asiatic calm," or "heavenly equanimity"), and massage it downward. The point is located directly under the tip of your ring finger when you place the inside of your hand across the kneecap. (See photo.)

Do not get discouraged if acupressure against your depressed mood does not succeed overnight, but keep on massaging each point for ten seconds (about thirty massage strokes per point) mornings, evenings, and, if need be, at noon. Do not omit *on your own* any of the antidepressants prescribed by your physician, but slowly reduce your drug intake only after consultation with your doctor.

DO YOU EAT MAINLY AFTER STRESS?

Check off:

yes no I wish I were more thick-skinned.

yes no I cannot go to work any longer without having taken a tranquilizer.

yes no I feel the aftereffects of conspicuous stress for several days.

yes no At times I am so irritable that no one can speak to me.

yes no I blow up easily.

yes no My co-workers sometimes say to me, "You need a vacation."

yes no But I am nervous during vacations, too.

If you have checked any of the statements with "yes," your handling of stress is out of proportion to the cause. You should be examined by a doctor, and after consultation with him, you should use the *shao-chong* acupressure point, always on both your left and right sides.

The next Chinese main point is the *ho-ku*, two finger widths below the knuckle at the base of the index finger and half a finger width toward the thumb. Massage it in the direction of the elbow, especially when you are exhausted through overexertion. The *lieh-ch'ueh* ("past the straits")

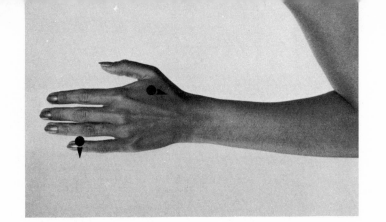

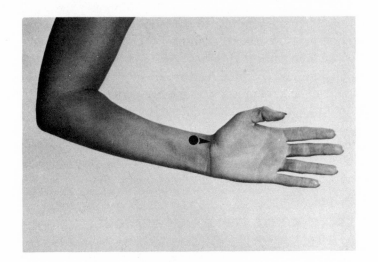

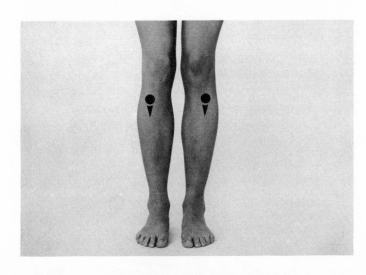

serves as the main point against all feelings of feebleness; it is located on the underside of the arm, two finger widths from the hand, at the spot where a doctor usually checks the pulse. Acupress it in the direction of the thumb.

Sometimes we get exhausted because, as a result of nervousness and lack of time, we take on too many things at once instead of "everything in its own good time." In such a situation, the point *tsu-san-li* helps one along. It can be found by placing the inside of the hand across the kneecap, with the tip of the middle finger reaching the shinbone; the point is then exactly under the tip of the ring finger, and has to be massaged in a downward motion.

Get enough sleep; abstain, especially when under stress, from alcohol and nicotine; and try to relax, at least on weekends and during vacations, preferably away from your usual surroundings for a complete change of scenery.

Massage each point one to three times daily, as needed, for about ten seconds (about thirty or more strokes per point). The antistress acupressure is used after the overeater's acupressure point (on the inside of the lower lip).

DO YOU OVEREAT FOR OTHER REASONS?

The overeater's acupressure on the point at the inside of the upper lip is necessary no matter what is the reason for your having become a compulsive eater, but it *is* important to recognize the cause. The cause may lie in the past and may have been removed, yet the aftereffects, in the form of overeating, linger on. Such was the case of Rose Lawler, a twenty-two-year-old patient, who had been jilted by her boyfriend. She began to overeat to overcome her frustration. Later on, when she had another boyfriend with whom she got along splendidly, she retained her unhealthy eating habits. It is easy to see that, in her case, the overeater's acupressure alone was enough, because the original cause of overeating had been removed.

The case of Henry Morris (thirty-one years old) is representative of many other patients. He is an engineer, and he told me in his businesslike manner: "The debit level of my satiety feeling has shifted upward." At fault was his mother, who had always put too much food on his plate, telling herself, "I want my child to be better off than I was." Henry's mother had, indeed, suffered real hardships in her youth; she had known real hunger, and had only seldom had a meat dish. Now, she wanted to make up for this with her son, and unfortunately always insisted that Henry clean his plate.

The result: Henry, five feet ten inches tall, had acquired faulty eating habits and weighed 202 pounds. In his case, too, the overeater's acupressure was sufficient, since Henry realized the cause, namely having been taught wrong eating habits. Henry practiced the overeater's acupressure and was able to change his eating habits. He has now reached what is for him the ideal weight of 162 pounds.

What can we learn from Rose Lawler and Henry Morris? In addition to the overeater's acupressure, it is essential to know the cause for the excessive eating and the resulting overweight. This cause then has to be eliminated. If you have a boss whose constant faultfinding drives you to compensate by overeating, I advise you to consider exchanging your job for one with more pleasant working conditions. Or, if your sailing companions are the ones who tempt you to drink too much, avoid their company, join a tennis club instead, and look there for partners who are less devoted to imbibing.

ACUPRESSURE: THE METHOD FOR EVERYONE

I am frequently asked whether everyone can use the overeater's acupressure with expectations of success. The answer is yes—any person who is overweight and is willing to use his brain. Everybody has, in fact, a feeding center in the brain that reacts to reflexes. When an overweight person sees a tempting dish, for instance, a stimulus immediately reaches his midbrain and he gets an appetite. If that person now applies the overeater's acupressure, the rule that the last stimulus erases the preceding one will hold true. The appetite is restrained, and this is done for everyone who correctly applies acupressure.

The degree of the restraint may vary. In one person the feeding center may be lastingly overstimulated to such an extent that the patient notices nothing on the first day of acupressure; the restraining effect is still too weak. If, in such an extreme case, the patient applies acupressure more frequently and longer than three times a day for ten seconds, and if the pressure is not too weak, the reflexes will become conditioned amazingly fast and the appetite, in fact, will disappear. In severe cases of overeating, until the acupressure begins to have an effect, this transition phase may last several days. That is normal. After a while, daily acupressure will have habituated the reflex pathways and you will be able to ease up on the pressure, shorten the time, and cut down on the number of daily massages.

If you follow the procedures suggested to you in this book, including the various diets, you will notice that the time required for acupressure decreases steadily. In fact, I know several patients who very successfully curb their appetite with only three to five seconds of acupressure before each meal. Such a patient should not apply acupressure longer than necessary. Just as the normal regulatory feeding center was turned into a compulsive-eating center by too much stimulation, the compulsive-eating center can be turned back into a well-functioning regulatory feeding center by restraining influences— namely the overeater's acupressure. This regulatory center will now tell us promptly when we should stop eating. This is what I want my method to accomplish for overweight readers: to restore the compulsive-eating center to a correctly functioning regulatory center.

Dangers of Acupressure: None

DANGERS FROM EXCESSIVE OR
NEUROTIC USE OF ACUPRESSURE

The use of acupressure is not accompanied by any dangers. However, if a physician has diagnosed neurotic behavior in someone, that patient should not use my method. Medical science has found that in neurotics, overeating can change into its opposite, a complete lack of appetite (*anorexia nervosa*). I would not want my method to be misused by inappropriate application—for example, someone continuing with the massage *after* the compulsive-eating center has already become a well-functioning feeding regulator. If that were done for any length of time, the continuous curbing of the reflexes could lead to a complete rejection of food. That too is an illness, and a physician, therefore, has to ascertain in advance whether a tendency to neurosis exists.

As a rule, all excesses are harmful. I consider it senseless if someone twenty or thirty pounds overweight starves herself into a skeleton to compete with the most emaciated fashion model. Such a radical change is, of course, damaging to health.

Our body is a nearly perfect machine. Yet, it needs time to readjust. If you want to lose a lot of weight, don't do it all at once. Reduce at first, under medical supervision, by ten to, at the most, twenty pounds. Remain on this plateau for about two to three months; just take care not to regain weight during that period. Only when your doctor tells you that your body has become adjusted should you go on losing another ten pounds. Then once more take a period for adjustment, and so forth.

AND NOW: THE DIET

Diet alone does not help, as we have ascertained; it removes the pounds but not the craving for food. Conversely, acupressure eliminates the craving but not the pounds, especially not the excess pounds present (later on, of course, it prevents the accumulation of new overweight). To reduce—made easy by acupressure—you need a diet. Which one?

To begin with, I assume that among my readers there are many who have tried once or several times to bring their weight down by dieting. If they were successful in shedding the desired number of pounds, without complications and harmful side effects, then, no matter what the diet, they did the right thing. It is not their fault that the unchanged, over-active feeding center later spoiled the effect.

If you have experience with dieting, you should combine a diet that you are familiar with and tolerated well with acupressure, and you will be successful. Only it will be much easier now; the self-control and self-denial that have always been necessary to stick to a reducing diet are no longer required, thanks to acupressure.

If you follow your own diet and do not want to use the regimens suggested by me (page 58, 250–300-calorie diet, page 65, 800-calorie diet, page 93, 1,300-calorie diet) you still have to keep in mind certain ground rules:

1) THE OVEREATER'S ACUPRESSURE

Before every meal apply the overeater's acupressure for ten seconds (for a little longer during the first days if necessary).

2) BEFORE EVERY MEAL HAVE SOMETHING TO DRINK

A glass of mineral water or low-calorie vegetable juice, sipped slowly before a meal, is filling and will further cut the appetite. During the meal, do not use the drink to wash down half-chewed bites.

3) CREATE A FEELING OF FULLNESS

Start every meal with a filler of low-calorie uncooked food, like a green salad, radishes, tomatoes, green peppers, carrots. Stuffing your stomach with noncaloric roughage will add to the effect of the overeater's acupressure in curbing the overactive feeding center.

4) EAT SLOWLY

Devote plenty of time to the introductory salad bowl. It takes a while until the body reacts to food intake; hunger only recedes about twenty minutes after the start of a meal. Whoever manages to wolf down a giant serving of pot roast and boiled potatoes in ten minutes will still be hungry and will clamor for more. But the person who leisurely consumes a large, tasty helping of cucumber salad, and takes his own good time doing it, will have stopped being hungry before he can eat more.

5) KEEP SMALL BETWEEN-MEALS SNACKS READY

Place a bowl of low-fat cottage cheese, together with a spoon, next to or in the refrigerator; or, if you prefer, substitute a plate of tomato salad or some cleaned radishes or celery. The chances are good that you will reach for these snacks instead of fetching a calorie bomb from the refrigerator.

6) TAKE SMALLER HELPINGS

It is recommended that your meals be served in suitably small portions, and no temptingly steaming serving bowls be placed on the dining table, especially after you have reached your desired weight through acupressure plus diet. You don't have to go so far as to eat exclusively from dessert plates, with teaspoons and dessert forks, as has been quite seriously suggested in many diet books. On the other hand, it isn't necessary to create additional temptations for yourself.

7) DON'T GO TO THE SUPERMARKET HUNGRY

Experience has shown that, while hungry, we reach for those foods that we like best; we don't consume them on the spot, but at home they will be a constant temptation once the food is within easy reach in the refrigerator.

8) SHOP WISELY

The decision whether you will eat too much, or buy the wrong food, is already being made while you are shopping. There is an enormous difference between a lean liverwurst and a German salami. Most packaged foods are labeled now as to content of carbohydrates, protein, fat, and calories; make use of these tables to select the product lower in calories, fat, and carbohydrates, and richer in protein.

A great number of high-quality foods with few calories (often designated as diabetic foods) can be bought not only in health food stores, but at most supermarkets. The low-calorie foods range from bread to sugar-free fruit juices and diet beer. These useful, special foods are somewhat more expensive than the regular ones, but since one eats significantly less, the extra expense will hardly affect your budget.

9) AVOID THE MISGUIDED ATTITUDE "NO LEFTOVERS"

For many overweight people, eating out presents a real problem. Employee cafeterias hardly ever offer suitable diet menus, and restaurants only seldom. And then there are those who, for the sake of their company, have to overeat: the whole range of salesmen and buyers, from the lowliest to the executives, who have to wine and dine their customers or partners. They march their usually already-too-impressive girths, in a companionable spirit, to the best restaurant in town and order whatever is good and expensive.

The importance of finishing up every last morsel is urged on us everywhere, in cafeterias, restaurants, and at home. Even children are familiar with the saying: "Waste not, want not." In someone fighting against overweight, such self-destructive avarice borders on idiocy.

In practice, you should eat only as much as you need, and

leave the rest on your plate without feeling embarrassed. Leftovers always mean calories not consumed. Tender souls affected by the sad face of the cook are free to let the culinary artist know how wonderfully tasty was the little they ate.

At a party in a private home it is more difficult to disappoint, or even offend, the hostess, especially when the food offered has been prepared with great care and effort by her own hands. In such cases you have to say "My doctor does not permit me to eat this"; or you have to invent, if necessary, an upset stomach. These excuses are always accepted, be it at a business lunch or at a family gathering in honor of a rich old uncle. No one expects you to eat something that might do you harm. And you are saved, by acupressure, from having to cast covetous glances at the other guests' plates.

CRASH DIETS ARE NOT NECESSARY

The temptation is certainly great to combine acupressure with a fast-working, frenzied crash diet. I disapprove.

The most extreme of all diets is doubtless fasting. I would not consider this a sensible procedure to follow. The end result is the same as with other diets, which means that the relapse quota is also usually about 85 percent. In addition, the complete cessation of any calorie intake often leads to disagreeable complications. These are so serious that a medical journal headed its summary of some lectures on fasting delivered at the 1977 Congress of German Internists with the impressive title: "Mortal Dangers Accompany Fasting." Recently a French reducing clinic extensively employing fasting had to close down because of several deaths.

Fasting is contraindicated for people suffering from liver disease or kidney disease, or from arteriosclerosis, and is not to be used in such cases. Obese people, especially older ones, often have problems with their liver, kidneys, or arteries. Moreover, fasting inevitably leads to muscle-tissue breakdown, since the body, deprived of all outside nourishment, resorts to "feeding itself from within" by consuming not only its own fat reserves, but also its muscle tissue. It even demolishes the heart muscle, in what is clearly an extremely dangerous effect.

All of this makes it doubtful whether fasting justifies all the effort and the expense for a hospital bed and medical supervision. To recommend use of fasting at home, something regrettably still being done, is totally irresponsible. A combination of acupressure and fasting is, therefore, out of the question.

EVERYTHING SLIMS YOU DOWN!

I also count among the extreme diets the one-sided programs; while unquestionably effective, they are anything but commendable. The confusion on this subject is correctly and entertainingly described in a mocking comment that appeared on October 8, 1977, in the *Süddeutsche Zeitung*. I reproduce it here in its entirety with permission by the author, Helmut Seitz:

> The other day, I was shopping at our butcher's. Two slices of pork loin, half a pound of cold cuts, and a bottle of red wine. (Lately, our butcher also carries frozen vegetables, canned fish, and even alcoholic beverages). Mr. Throwbones beat the meat slices, weighed the cold cuts, wrapped the wine, and handed me everything across the counter, together with a copy of *Cutlet,* that great periodical for the customers of the butcher's trade. For my entertainment, said Mr. Throwbones, and as a reminder to come again.
>
> The contents of this sheet were not what I would call exciting: a short story, a crossword puzzle, a piece of a serial novel, and a handful of tips for the housewife. Ah, but wait! There was something very interesting on page two. A highly scientific essay with the promising title, "Get Slim While Eating to Your Heart's Content." This article stated plainly and simply that there is only one way to become slim without starvation diets. One only has to eat meat and sausages, the more the better. Meat products for breakfast, meat for lunch, meat for dinner, and meat in between.

For meat satisfies, meat is slimming, meat contains vital protein, meat gives strength, and meat always tastes good!

The other day, I shopped at our baker's. Six seeded rolls, a whole-grain bread, and a reference work, on special sale at a good price. (Lately, our baker carries, in addition to eggs, butter, and coffee, also books.) Mrs. Doughtwist handed me, free of charge, a copy of *Our Daily Bread,* the great publication for the customers of the baker's trade. To entertain me, and to make me come again. This paper, too, contained the usual: a short story, an installment of the unavoidable novel, a crossword puzzle, and traditional recipes for the housewife. Ah, but wait! There, on page three, something interesting: a highly scientific essay with the promising title, "Slim down without fasting." This article proved that you have to eat bread, bread, and more bread, for bread satisfies but is not fattening. Moreover, bread contains vital body-building ingredients, and any number of vitamins. Bread is also healthful. Therefore, you should cut thicker slices and go easy on the calorie-rich spreads! In addition, bread always tastes good and offers so much variety.

The other day, I shopped at our vegetable store: a head of lettuce, oranges, and a tube of toothpaste. The store lately carries cosmetics in addition to newspapers, cigarettes, and bottled beer. Mr. Coleslaw also presented me with a magazine for customers, and there I found, next to a short story, the obligatory recipes, and the installment of a novel, an interesting article with the intriguing title, "Stay healthy, slim down, yet want for nothing!" Ever since, I know that all one has to do is eat fruit and vegetables, as much fresh fruit and vegetables as possible. For fruit and vegetables are healthy, fruit and vegetables are living food, fruit and vegetables always taste good and do not overload the body with unnecessary ballast. Fruit and vegetables! Vegetables and fruit!

From other sources I also learned that fish does not make you fat. And milk, butter, and cheese, even less—not to speak of nourishing and easily digested eggs. If you want to stay slim, slim and healthy, all you have to do is eat plenty of meat, sausages, eggs, fish, cheese, bread, fruit, vegetables, and butter. Of course, also lots of rice and potatoes and don't stint on noodles and desserts. Because, as you have been told, nothing makes you fat, everything is slimming, if only you eat enough of it. Since most people follow this advice anyway, where do all those extra pounds come from? Most definitely not from eating, claims not only every one of the trade papers, but swears every fat person upon his or her solemn oath.

Strange as it may sound, taken singly, all these claims are correct. If you eat meat, meat, and nothing but meat, you will eventually lose weight. After eating only steaks, cutlets, and London broil, you will get so tired of it that you will not want to eat much, and will, in effect, consume considerably fewer calories.

The same holds true for only eggs, eggs, eggs; or only rolls, rolls, rolls; or only potatoes, potatoes, potatoes. The only trouble is that none of these methods is healthful. Another recently developed variation, the egg-and-whiskey diet, no doubt attractive for the heavy drinker, cannot possibly claim to be healthful either.

The method of cutting down on calories by simply skipping a meal has just as little to recommend it. When too much time passes between meals, blood-sugar level, as well as blood pressure, falls below the normal; dizziness, cold sweat, heart palpitation, even fainting can be the result, and longer reaction time could become dangerous in traffic. Especially if one skips breakfast can one expect such consequences. Such methods may be quick, but they make you sick.

In summary, acupressure, which frees you from compulsion, should not be combined with extreme or fad diets. Most of these diets aim for a very quick weight loss, mainly to shorten the time of painful renunciation. But if you phase out your craving for food through acupressure, eating less than before does not make you suffer. For this reason, it is not necessary to brutally force your body to give up its excess pounds.

In combination with acupressure, you should adopt a well-balanced, gentle diet that causes the body, without overtaxing it, to break down its fat. Too quick a weight loss also causes esthetic problems. The skin cannot contract fast enough to keep up with shrinking flesh; the connective tissue under the skin loses its fat; and the skin becomes slack. This is not attractive, especially on your face.

WHAT DOES THE BODY NEED?
WHAT CAN IT DO WITHOUT?

1) INDISPENSABLE: PROTEIN

Protein occurs in prodigious variety; it is the basis of all living substances. Each individual cell—the human body consists of about 6 trillion cells—contains protein. During our entire lifetime, every single second, billions of cells become useless, die, are cast off or eliminated, and have to be replaced by new ones. The body, therefore, needs constant replacement of protein, the building material for its cells. Hormones and enzymes also consist of highly complex molecules that the body builds out of simple protein components. The daily minimum requirement of protein is one to two grams per two pounds of body weight (variable according to sex and age), and the body should not be deprived of it under any circumstances; an average supply of two and one half to three ounces daily is, therefore, needed by the average person.

Because each species of plant and animal possesses its own unique set of proteins, man cannot utilize directly the proteins he consumes in animal or plant foods. Instead, his body must transform the food into suitable proteins. Man's protein needs are best served by food that consists of half animal protein, half plant protein.

High-grade animal protein is available from milk, especially fat-free milk, buttermilk, curdled milk, yogurt (be sure to get unsweetened yogurt without fruit), cottage cheese, and cheese; also in fish, meat, and eggs. Plant protein is contained in practically every vegetarian food, especially in grain products, potatoes, vegetables, and legumes—particularly in soybeans.

2) TEMPORARILY DISPENSABLE: CARBOHYDRATES

Carbohydrates is the chemical catchall term for starch and sugar. They are the main suppliers of energy for the organism; with their help, the whole complicated machinery is kept running. Excess carbohydrates, stored as reserves, are transformed into fat, since large amounts of energy are best stored, over any length of time, in the form of fat. When the body has to call on its stored energy, it changes the fat back into carbohydrates. For this reason, it is not only feasible, but essential for weight reduction, to restrict the carbohydrate intake as much as possible; this causes the body to live on its own stored fat and, thereby, to break down the unsightly bulges.

Carbohydrates are plentiful in bread, including whole-grain and rye bread; in all cereal products like rice, semolina, oatmeal, etc.; in fruit (fruit sugar!); vegetables; potatoes; and, of course, in sugar, honey, and sweets of all kinds. A veritable super-carbohydrate is alcohol, an energy carrier whose role in overweight is often underestimated by those affected.

3) ALMOST WHOLLY DISPENSABLE: FAT

The body needs a substantial supply of fat only when required to perform heavy labor. A lumberman using an ax can well tolerate a good chunk of bacon for his second breakfast; during such high energy expenditure, fat is virtually not stored at all, but is immediately converted into energy. On the other hand, a man who already has too much stored fat on his body and is unable to use it up by physical exertion needs hardly any additional fat.

But fat does not only serve the energy supply, it also acts as a solvent for some important vitamins. The body fat is of no use here, since it is not in the stomach or intestines, but in those conspicuous storage areas. For this reason, a certain amount of fat must be part of what you eat, to channel the vitamins, ingested together with food, into the body's house-

hold, instead of eliminating them, unused, through the digestive system. The body also needs, in small quantities, certain
fatty acids—linoleic acid, for instance.

The total amount of fat needed is very small—only frac-
tions of an ounce per day—and those are, in any case, contained as so-called "hidden fats" in other foods that do not
appear to be fatty at all. One egg, for instance, contains about
two tenths of an ounce of fat; a pint of milk, half an ounce;
a small, three-and-a-half ounce, lean cutlet, prepared without
fat, half an ounce.

4) INDISPENSABLE: VITAMINS AND MINERALS

Without an adequate supply of vitamins, which have various
protecting, regulating, and stimulating functions, one inevitably gets sick. A sufficient supply of minerals that are needed
as building blocks, is also indispensable. Calcium, for instance,
is necessary for healthy bones; potassium is needed to prevent
irregularities of the heart rhythm.

Vitamins and minerals are usually adequately represented
in normal food intake, but during a diet may decrease below
a critical margin. To compensate, one should take multi-vita-
min tablets enriched with minerals, since fruit, because of its
fruit-sugar content (carbohydrate!) is not permitted in a strict
diet.

5) INDISPENSABLE WITH A SCANTY DIET: FILLERS

Diets, no matter which ones, cause a conspicuous reduction
in the quantity of food eaten, especially when the aim is fast
weight reduction. When the body is given only the necessary
minimum, little bulk is left, and this is a serious drawback
because stomach and intestines are underemployed. In practice, this means constipation; nothing moves along. Yet, a
functioning digestion is absolutely indispensable. This can be
achieved with the help of a whole range of quite well-liked
foods that hardly deserve the name "food," since they have

practically no nutritional value. They do have bulk, though, which is almost totally indigestible but which nevertheless leads the digestive system to make a try and, therefore, to keep going.

Such nearly calorie-free fillers, ballast, or fiber material are: cucumbers, radishes, cauliflower, celery, kohlrabi, peppers, lettuce, endives, watercress, carrots, broccoli, zucchini, tomatoes, and spinach. An important beneficial side effect is that nearly all these fillers, so important for the diet, also contain essential minerals and vitamins.

WHICH DIET WITH ACUPRESSURE?

If—aside from being overweight—you are in good health, you should start with a protein-and-raw-vegetable diet of from 250 to 300 calories, but only for one week or at the most two, and under medical supervision.

It is preferable not to start the regimen when you are carrying a maximum work load or are otherwise overextended. Although acupressure will save you from feeling starved, the changeover of the body from external to internal energy-supply (breaking down of fat) is still a process that should not be aggravated by additional burdens. The body, after all, will have to release daily 1,500 to 2,000 calories from its store of fat. And this is also the reason for the—admittedly—veritable jackrabbit start: The body should be forced to quickly readjust, and it needs a forceful send-off.

This starter diet is out of the question for people suffering from diabetes or gout, or for people with a propensity for kidney stones. As a matter of principle, the same holds true for this diet as for any other: All dieting requires readjustment of the body, and needs medical supervision.

THE IDEAL COMBINATION:

Ten seconds of the overeater's acupressure and a 250- to 300-calorie protein-and-raw-vegetable diet

BREAKFAST

(preceded by ten seconds of anti-compulsive-eating acupressure)
1 boiled egg, or a protein concentrate (E.M.F. or L.P.P.), or an unsweetened low-fat yogurt. Two to three cups of tea or coffee, without milk or sugar; if you like, use artificial sweetener. (If you have a craving for bread, first use anti-compulsive-eating acupressure, then put a piece of bread in your mouth, chew it only a little, and spit it out.)

MIDMORNING

2 glasses of tomato juice or vegetable juice.

LUNCH

(preceded by ten seconds of anti-compulsive-eating acupressure)
2 cups of unsweetened tea or 2 glasses of mineral water. A very large bowl of cucumber salad, or a lettuce salad, or coleslaw, made with a few spoons of low-fat yogurt and chives, or prepared with lemon juice and *only a few drops* of oil.

AFTERNOON

2 glasses of tomato juice, vegetable juice, or sauerkraut juice; or 1 cup of consommé or bouillion.

DINNER

(preceded by ten seconds of anti-compulsive-eating acupressure)
2–3 glasses of mineral water
5 ounces low-fat cottage cheese mixed with chives, tomatoes, green peppers, or radishes; or a protein concentrate (E.M.F. or L.P.P.); or 2 skim-milk yogurts (unsweetened, without fruit). *You must have:* some raw vegetables, like cucumber, radishes, tomatoes, celery, pepper, etc.

NOTE: Include no fruit, but instead multivitamin-plus-mineral tablets (to avoid fruit sugar).

Your daily totals are:
   2–3 quarts of liquid
   3–5 ounces of protein
   14–25 ounces of raw vegetables
   Hardly any fat or carbohydrates

To keep the cholesterol level low, you should eat not more than 3 or 4 eggs per week.

WHY IS THE COMBINATION OF PROTEIN AND RAW VEGETABLES SO IMPORTANT?

The Food and Drug Administration is planning to permit the sale of protein concentrates only if they carry a label with the warning that use of these preparations as *sole* nourishment could lead to "serious illness or death." If this warning does not seem to be sufficiently effective, the FDA, according to its director, Donald Kennedy, is considering requiring prescriptions to buy these protein concentrates.

The reason for these steps was the death of several dozen people who had been reducing without medical supervision for a long time, and had eaten nothing but the protein concentrates. They died of heart failure. Most likely, potassium deficiency was at fault, since potassium is a mineral absolutely essential for a steady heart rhythm. The FDA, according to press reports, believes that some of the protein concentrates may contain too little potassium. All this has confirmed my opinion that using protein concentrates as *sole* nourishment, no matter how convenient that may seem, is definitely not advisable. On the contrary, raw vegetables have to be added, since they are very rich in potassium and in general are rich in minerals and vitamins.

In the combination proposed by me, protein concentrates are certainly very useful, because the normal foods in a 250–

300-calorie diet simply cannot provide the necessary proteins. When there is a lack of proteins, the body immediately falls back upon its own reserves, foremost among them muscle protein, and that too is harmful. Herein lies one of the serious dangers of fasting, which of necessity leads to protein deficiency. You could and should use protein concentrates for a supplement, but not—and I repeat not—under any circumstances as sole nourishment.

KEEPING YOUR BOWELS FUNCTIONING

I strongly advise against restricting your diet solely to proteins out of a bottle, not only because of the danger of potassium deficiency, but because of the near certainty of trouble with the almost completely unemployed digestive system. The intestines have to be kept busy, which is also a reason why I recommend the protein-and-raw-vegetables combination. The raw vegetables consist of ballast materials, to a large extent. These keep the bowels functioning well.

WHY MULTIVITAMIN TABLETS INSTEAD OF FRUIT DURING THE STARTER DIET?

The indicated 250–300-calorie daily ration cannot contain all the vitamins in sufficient quantities, since fruits have to be avoided because of their high fruit-sugar (carbohydrate) content. Therefore, you have to take a supplementary multivitamin tablet, preferably one enriched with minerals, so that the body can absorb the fat-soluble vitamins. Our diet is not totally, but only almost, fat-free; the eggs and cottage cheese and the few drops of oil in your salad contain the necessary small quantity of fat.

It is obvious that the starter diet cannot allow for great variety. Of course, it doesn't have to be cucumber salad every day; Boston lettuce or endive is just as good. If you don't like the yogurt dressing, use vinegar or lemon. With this, you can use a few drops of oil (but truly only a few drops). If you don't like to have an egg for breakfast, substitute a container of unsweetened low-fat yogurt (without fruit).

The addition of half a small chopped onion, or radishes, chives, or paprika to improve the taste of salads and of cottage cheese is gladly permitted. Some people like their cottage cheese sweet; for them there are liquid artificial sweeteners.

It is important to drink as much as possible, even more than the indicated quantities. Drinking two to three quarts of liquid a day is by no means excessive. It isn't all that easy to get such quantities down, however. It is advisable, therefore, to always have a glass of mineral water, tomato juice, or vegetable juice (no fruit juice) within easy reach during this time. This will prompt you to take a drink. There may be a few exceptions as far as the fruit juices are concerned: A grapefruit juice with little sugar content has been on the market lately. There are also tasty diet lemonades with fewer than twenty calories per glass.

You may drink a lot of tomato juice (however, this is not good for people prone to develop kidney stones, since tomato juice is rich in calcium). Tomato juice has few calories and the body has to use up a certain amount of energy to digest the juice, which means that calories are being spent. If you deduct these calories from the ones in the tomato juice, not much is left.

NECESSARY: BLOOD-PRESSURE CHECKS

Before you start your diet, a physician has to check your blood pressure. Normally, blood pressure decreases during the diet—which in many cases is desirable, since *most overweight people's blood pressure is too high*. Blood pressure has to be checked during the diet, as it should not be permitted to fall so low as to cause dizziness or fainting. Plenty of liquids and enough salt (for instance, salt the tomato juice, the cucumber salad, etc.) are usually sufficient to keep the blood pressure stable. If you had been taking medicines for high blood pressure, your doctor may now want to reduce the dosage. But if you already had low blood pressure, you may need a circulatory drug in addition to plentiful liquids and salt. In each case, blood-pressure checks by a doctor are necessary.

YES! YOU MADE IT! YOU ARE RID OF THE FIRST FEW POUNDS!

Now you are on your way! If you began the acupressure diet combination with the skimpy protein-and-raw-vegetable diet, you are weighing quite a bit less by now. Depending on your initial weight and the time you stayed with the starter diet, you lost between five and thirteen pounds.

If, for health reasons, you were unable to begin with the 250–300-calorie diet, or chose not to do so—for the reason, perhaps, that you had only a little weight to lose—then start with the following diet. It is calculated to provide about 800 calories per day and guarantees you a steady, effective weight loss.

The diet has been calculated for you, which means *you do not have to calculate*. It takes all the fun out of eating, I think, if you have to keep a calorie table and a slide rule or pocket computer next to your plate. That should not be necessary and, anyway, who would use them consistently and correctly?

Anyway, the usual procedure is to eat first and then count the calories; in most cases there will be too many. To compensate, an entire meal may then be skipped, and the result is unhealthful, because the interval between meals is too long. I prefer to offer you daily menus that you know contain the desired 800 calories, sensibly distributed over the day. Please turn to the daily menus starting on page 67 to see what I mean.

You do not have to adhere slavishly to the daily grouping. If you particularly like two or three of the breakfast suggestions, there is no reason why you should not stay with them. Many people eat the same breakfast, day in and day out; this may be boring but does no harm as long as the breakfast consists of the right foods. The morning meals suggested here have about 250 calories each.

The low-calorie between-meals suggestions may present problems for some people. It generally—and regrettably—has become the custom to have only three meals a day. Even under normal conditions this isn't good; during the long interval between meals, the blood-sugar level and often the blood pressure sink, and productivity decreases. It decreases once more after a meal which, if it is one of only three, will have to be fairly substantial. The body concentrates on digesting the food; more blood goes to the stomach and intestines, proportionally less to the head; brain activity slows (that causes the tired feeling that regularly overcomes us after a plentiful meal).

What is not good under normal circumstances is even less desirable during a reducing diet. Therefore, grant your body the in-between meals. While you are dieting, you want to— and should—remain fully productive. You should not eat less than those scant 800 calories; it is just the right amount to assure you of trouble-free well-being and simultaneous breakdown of fat, over a period of time.

How much fat does the body break down during an 800-calorie diet? You can easily calculate that: In three and a half ounces of body fat, as it collects, for instance, on the hips, energy corresponding to 930 calories is stored. If you reduce the daily food intake of about 2,600 calories (a moderate estimate for overweight people) to 800, about 1,800 calories are missing; these must be replaced from stored fat. To do this, the body has to break down seven ounces of fat, which means that you will lose almost half a pound per day with this diet; almost two pounds in four days; thirteen pounds in one month. If you start with a lot of overweight, you will even lose a bit more.

BEVERAGES

During this stage you should also drink as much as possible; choose no fruit juices containing a lot of sugar, but instead, drink the already-mentioned low-calorie thirst-quenchers.

Alcohol is out! You have to realize that alcohol cancels out the effects of any diet. The reason is plain. Alcohol is an outstanding storer of energy and, at the same time, is closely related to fat chemically: Fats are formed by combining alcohol with fatty acids, and our body is highly skilled in this technique. After having made a nuisance of itself in the liver, the alcohol is promptly converted into the finest fat, and lots of it, since alcohol is incredibly rich in energy. For this reason the volume of fat formed from alcohol is correspondingly large. If you seriously want to get rid of your overweight, you have to avoid alcohol in any form. One of the reasons is that a considerable number of overweight people largely owe the "over" that they would and should shed, to customary social drinking.

A few hints: If you find it too difficult to stick to the alcohol prohibition, drink at the most one bottle of the kind of diet beer developed for diabetics. It contains few carbohydrates and hardly any alcohol. One glass of a very dry white wine with your dinner won't tip the energy balance. And one more trick: A dash of light red wine in a glass of mineral water makes the latter look friendlier and taste better, and hardly adds to the calories.

THE 800-CALORIE DIET: RECIPES

As you start the 800-calorie diet you must understand that the few foods that are expected to keep you fully productive have to be of the best quality. For instance, fruit and vegetables have to be fresh and, as far as possible, uncooked; the oil should be from the first pressing—that is, it should have been pressed cold; instead of white bread, choose whole-wheat bread. Just as important as the well-chosen quality is the right preparation. Instead of roasting and frying, you should boil, steam, broil, or cook in aluminum foil.

As you contemplate the small size of the indicated model

meals, you may have the bright idea to simply throw in an all-fruit day instead. I warn you! You are underrating the high calorie count of fruit sugar. (One pound of fruit has an average of 250 calories.) It certainly won't do you any harm to slip in, here and there, a day of eating only raw vegetables. That is not the same as a day of just fruit! But I cannot stress enough how important a factor *variety* is—especially during reduced food intake—to avoid deficiency diseases that would be added to the damage already done by false eating habits.

To live with this reducing diet, you will be supported by anti-compulsive-eating acupressure, but also by a certain artistry: The food has to be appetizing without giving you an appetite! The spartan 800 calories do not give you much scope, but there is no need for the kind of monotony experienced with the liquid-protein diet, which is seen as self-punishment by many overweight people, and for that reason as unacceptable.

The daily 800 calories also cannot accommodate all the necessary proteins and vitamins you need—at least not for certain individual requirements. Depending on personal needs, supplementary protein concentrates and multivitamins enriched with minerals should be taken, preferably in the evening, during this reducing phase.

And now let us start out on a few weeks of our 800-calorie diet, which is poor in fats and carbohydrates. Each and every day you should lose about half a pound. For this diet, as for any other, medical supervision is indispensable, since *all* diets require readjustment of body functions. Medical control is especially necessary in the case of patients suffering from liver or kidney trouble, or from heart or circulatory diseases. Neither should this diet be used during pregnancy; only after the child is born can the overweight be reduced.

If a restaurant visit or an unavoidable party at a friend's house caused you to eat, one day, more than the allotted 800 calories, you can make up for this by one day of our 300-calorie starter regimen.

DAY 1

BREAKFAST
*(preceded by ten seconds of
anti-compulsive-eating acupressure):*

1 slice mixed-grain bread
1 egg
1 tomato
Tea or coffee, with milk, if you prefer, but without sugar
(sweeten to taste with artificial sweetener)

IN-BETWEEN MEAL

7 ounces of strawberries or raspberries, without sugar

LUNCH
*(preceded by ten seconds of
anti-compulsive-eating acupressure):*
VEAL CUTLET AND GREEN SALAD

4½ ounces veal cutlet
Salt, paprika, pepper
1 small onion
1 scant teaspoon oil, a little vinegar, spices
2 small potatoes

Season the meat with salt and paprika, and sauté it in a
coated pan, without fat. Trim the salad greens, wash them,
and make a dressing of vinegar, oil, the small onion, salt,
pepper, and spices. Serve with the two small boiled potatoes.

IN-BETWEEN MEAL

1 glass tomato juice

DINNER
*(preceded by ten seconds of
anti-compulsive-eating acupressure):*

1 glass buttermilk (8 ounces)
1 ounce soft cheese
1 thin piece of dark pumpernickel
1 green salad

D A Y   2

800 calories

BREAKFAST
*(preceded by ten seconds of the
overeater's acupressure):*

1 glass freshly squeezed orange juice
2 thin slices of dark pumpernickel
½ ounce of lean liverwurst
Tea or coffee, with milk, if you prefer (sweeten to taste with
artificial sweetener)

IN-BETWEEN MEAL

1 apple (5 ounces)

LUNCH
*(preceded by ten seconds of the
overeater's acupressure):*

FILET MIGNON WITH CAULIFLOWER FLOWERETTES

4 ounces filet mignon
7 ounces cauliflower
½ tsp butter
1 tsp oil
¾ ounce instant mashed potatoes
1 tbsp milk, 1 tbsp water
Salt, nutmeg, pepper

Rub filet with oil, sprinkle with salt and pepper, and sauté in
hot pan. Boil the cauliflower flowerettes in salted water until
barely tender; season with nutmeg. Bring milk and water to

a boil together with the butter; stir in the instant mashed potatoes; season to taste with salt and nutmeg.

IN-BETWEEN MEAL

1 glass grapefruit juice (without sugar)

DINNER
*(preceded by ten seconds of the
overeater's acupressure):*

2 pieces of rye crisp
2 ounces (4 slices) smoked ham
1 tomato

DAY 3

800 calories

BREAKFAST
*(preceded by ten seconds of the
overeater's acupressure):*

1 slice rye bread
3½ ounces of low-fat cottage cheese
1 tomato
Tea or coffee, with milk, if you prefer (sweeten to taste with artificial sweetener)

IN-BETWEEN MEAL

1 large peach (5 ounces)

LUNCH
*(preceded by ten seconds of the
overeater's acupressure):*
POACHED TROUT AND GREEN SALAD

1 trout (9 ounces)
2 small potatoes
5 ounces salad greens
3 tbsp low-fat yogurt
Vinegar or lemon juice, salt, dill, parsley
½ ounce butter

Wash the trout, dry it, sprinkle it with lemon juice or vinegar, permit it to stand for a half hour, dry it again, salt it inside and out. Place it in a pan with 1½ quarts of boiling salted water; turn heat down immediately and simmer for about 20 minutes. Brown the butter, add chopped parsley and pour the mixture over the fish and the boiled potatoes. For the salad use a dressing of 3 tbsp low-fat yogurt, salt, pepper, and dill.

IN-BETWEEN MEAL

1 apple

DINNER
(preceded by ten seconds of the overeater's acupressure):

1 scrambled egg with chives
1 slice of toast
Radishes

DAY 4

800 calories

BREAKFAST
(preceded by ten seconds of the overeater's acupressure):

1 slice of graham bread
2 slices of smoked ham
1 glass tomato juice
Tea or coffee, with milk, if you prefer (sweeten to taste with artificial sweetener)

IN-BETWEEN MEAL

1 container low-fat yogurt

LUNCH
*(preceded by ten seconds of the
overeater's acupressure):*
CANNED MUSHROOMS WITH MASHED POTATOES

 9 ounces canned mushrooms
½ ounce butter
1¾ ounces instant mashed potatoes
 1 tbsp milk, 1 tbsp water
 1 small onion, parsley, salt, pepper, nutmeg

Drain the mushrooms. Heat the butter in a coated pan, sauté onion until transparent, add the mushrooms, and heat. Season with salt, pepper, and minced fresh parsley. Serve with mashed potatoes (see Day 2).

IN-BETWEEN MEAL
3½ ounces buttermilk

DINNER
*(preceded by ten seconds of the
overeater's acupressure):*

 1 slice whole-wheat bread
½ ounce lean liverwurst
 1 tomato

DAY 5

800 calories

BREAKFAST
*(preceded by ten seconds of the
overeater's acupressure):*

1 grapefruit (without sugar)
2 thin slices of pumpernickel
4 slices filet of smoked ham
Tea or coffee, with milk, if you prefer (sweeten to taste with artificial sweetener)

IN-BETWEEN MEAL
1 cup clear instant broth

LUNCH
(preceded by ten seconds of the
overeater's acupressure):
SPINACH AND FRIED EGG

9 ounces spinach
½ ounce butter or margarine
1 small onion, salt
1 egg
2 small potatoes

Melt butter or margarine in a skillet, sauté the chopped onion until transparent, add spinach, sauté briefly, run the mixture through the blender and season with salt and nutmeg. Serve with one egg, fried without fat, and the boiled potatoes.

IN-BETWEEN MEAL
1 cup clear instant broth

DINNER
(preceded by ten seconds of the
overeater's acupressure):
SHRIMP COCKTAIL

1 piece of rye crisp
Mix 3 ounces of boiled shrimp with a few cubes of pineapple, ½ a boiled egg and diet mayonnaise.

D A Y 6

800 calories

BREAKFAST
(preceded by ten seconds of the
overeater's acupressure):

1 slice mixed-grain bread
3½ ounces cottage cheese with chives, radishes
Tea or coffee, with milk, if you prefer (sweeten to taste with artificial sweetener)

IN-BETWEEN MEAL

1 cup clear instant broth

LUNCH
*(preceded by ten seconds of the
overeater's acupressure):*
CALF'S LIVER WITH MUSHROOMS, TOMATO SALAD,
AND RICE

5 ounces calf's liver
2 small onions, salt, curry powder, pepper
1 ounce mushrooms
2 tomatoes
½ ounce margarine
2 tbsp evaporated milk

Cut liver into strips and sauté together with one chopped onion in the margarine for 6–8 minutes. Don't salt liver before cooking—this hardens it. Add sliced mushrooms, then the evaporated milk, and simmer for another 5 minutes. Season with salt and a little pepper and curry powder. Slice tomatoes and sprinkle with salt, pepper, and 1 minced onion. Serve with 2 tbsp cooked rice.

IN-BETWEEN MEAL

1 low-fat yogurt

DINNER
*(preceded by ten seconds of the
overeater's acupressure):*
SHRIMP SALAD

7 ounces boiled shrimp
1 grated apple
2 tbsp cooked rice
Chopped onion, lemon juice
1 piece of rye crisp

DAY 7

800 calories

BREAKFAST
(preceded by ten seconds of the overeater's acupressure):

1 glass freshly squeezed orange juice
1 slice whole-grain bread
1 slice cold meat
1 tomato
Tea or coffee, with milk, if you prefer (sweeten to taste with artificial sweetener)

IN-BETWEEN MEAL

1 glass buttermilk
1 orange

LUNCH
(preceded by ten seconds of the overeater's acupressure):
POTATOES BOILED IN THEIR JACKETS, COTTAGE CHEESE, AND ENDIVE SALAD

2 small potatoes
4½ ounces low-fat cottage cheese
1 small onion, chives, salt
3½ ounces endives
3 tbsp skim milk

Season the cottage cheese with half the chopped onion, salt, and chives; cream it with the skim milk. Cut up the endives, wash them, and soak them for half an hour in lukewarm water. Drain the endives and season them with a dressing of 1 scant tbsp oil, vinegar, the remaining half onion, salt, pepper, and spices.

IN-BETWEEN MEAL

1 cup consommé or bouillion

DINNER
*(preceded by ten seconds of the
overeater's acupressure):*

1 thin slice of pumpernickel
2 slices smoked filet of ham
Carrot-celery-apple salad

Finely grate or chop 2 ounces carrots, 2 ounces celery, ½ apple. Mix with ½ tsp oil, lemon juice, and artificial sweetener.

DAY 8

800 calories

BREAKFAST
*(preceded by ten seconds of the
overeater's acupressure):*

2 tangerines
1 slice whole-grain bread with 1 ounce soft cheese
Tea or coffee, with milk, if you prefer (sweeten to taste with artificial sweetener)

IN-BETWEEN MEAL
9½ ounces of melon

LUNCH
*(preceded by ten seconds of the
overeater's acupressure):*
ROUND STEAK AND GARLIC BEANS, GREEN SALAD

4 ounces round steak
4½ ounces fresh green beans
Garlic, salt, pepper

Salt the steak, sprinkle it with pepper, and broil or grill it without fat. Boil the beans in 1 quart salted water or steam them (the latter method is better, because more vitamins are preserved). Drain the beans and season them with savory, garlic, salt. For salad: see Day 1.

IN-BETWEEN MEAL

1 cup clear instant broth

DINNER
(preceded by ten seconds of the
overeater's acupressure):

1 slice whole-grain bread
2 scrambled eggs with chives
2 tomatoes

DAY 9

800 calories

BREAKFAST
(preceded by ten seconds of the
overeater's acupressure):

1 low-fat yogurt
¾ ounce lean calf's liverwurst
2 pieces of rye crisp
Tea or coffee, with milk, if you prefer (sweeten to taste with
artificial sweetener)

IN-BETWEEN MEAL

2 apricots

LUNCH
(preceded by ten seconds of the
overeater's acupressure):
PORK CUTLET WITH KOHLRABI OR TURNIP;
CUCUMBER SALAD

3½ ounces pork cutlet
Salt, pepper, paprika, dill, parsley
1 small cucumber
1 kohlrabi or turnip
3 tbsp low-fat yogurt
½ ounce butter or margarine

Season cutlet with salt, pepper, and paprika and fry or grill it without fat. Pare and slice the kohlrabi or turnip, boil in salted water and drain. Melt butter or margarine in a skillet; add the kohlrabi; season it with salt, pepper, and spices. Sprinkle fresh minced parsley over the kohlrabi. For cucumber salad, prepare a dressing of low-fat yogurt, dill, salt, and pepper.

IN-BETWEEN MEAL

1 glass tomato juice

DINNER
(preceded by ten seconds of the
overeater's acupressure):

3½ ounces spiced low-fat cottage cheese, prepared by mixing with tomato, sour pickle, herbs, and spices
1 slice graham bread
Radishes

D A Y   1 0
800 calories

BREAKFAST
(preceded by ten seconds of the
overeater's acupressure):

½ grapefruit (without sugar)
2 slices toast
1 egg
Tea or coffee, with milk, if you prefer (sweeten to taste with artificial sweetener)

IN-BETWEEN MEAL

1 glass buttermilk

LUNCH
*(preceded by ten seconds of the
overeater's acupressure):*
BRAISED HEART OF VEAL

5 ounces heart of veal
A few drops of oil
1¾ ounces yogurt
3½ ounces potatoes
3½ ounces Boston lettuce

Fry heart of veal lightly in oil together with soup greens and
spices; add 1½ ounces yogurt to make a sauce. Serve with
potatoes and salad. Prepare dressing of 2 tbsp low-fat yogurt,
pepper, salt, and dill.

IN-BETWEEN MEAL

2 tangerines

DINNER
*(preceded by ten seconds of the
overeater's acupressure):*

1¾ ounces beefsteak tartare
1 thin slice of pumpernickel
Radishes

DAY 11

800 calories

BREAKFAST
*(preceded by ten seconds of the
overeater's acupressure):*

1 cup yogurt
2 whole-grain rusks
½ ounce honey
Tea or coffee, with milk, if you prefer (sweeten to taste with
artificial sweetener)

IN-BETWEEN MEAL

1 glass tomato juice
1 green pepper

LUNCH
*(preceded by ten seconds of the
overeater's acupressure):*
STEAMED PIKE, MASHED POTATOES, AND SALAD

10 ounces steamed pike
Prepare salad with dressing of lemon juice, a little chopped onion, various spices, and a few drops of oil. For mashed potatoes see Day 2.

IN-BETWEEN MEAL

1 peach

DINNER
*(preceded by ten seconds of the
overeater's acupressure):*
ASPARAGUS SALAD WITH BREAST OF CHICKEN

7 ounces asparagus
3½ ounces breast of chicken
1 piece of rye crisp

DAY 12

800 calories

BREAKFAST
*(preceded by ten seconds of the
overeater's acupressure):*

2 thin slices of pumpernickel
3½ ounces cottage cheese with herbs
2 tomatoes
Tea or coffee, with milk, if you prefer (sweeten to taste with artificial sweetener)

IN-BETWEEN MEAL

1 pear (5 ounces)

LUNCH
*(preceded by ten seconds of the
overeater's acupressure):*
RAGOUT OF ROAST CHICKEN WITH APPLE SALAD AND RICE

5 ounces of leftovers of roast chicken cubed in a sauce of
lemon juice, mustard, artificial sweetener, sautéd chopped
onion, and mushrooms. Serve with 2 tbsp rice. For the
salad, cube the apple and mix with a lot of lemon juice, a
few orange segments and some artificial sweetener.

IN-BETWEEN MEAL

2 tangerines
1 rusk

DINNER
*(preceded by ten seconds of the
overeater's acupressure):*

1 thin slice of pumpernickel
½ ounce lean calf's liverwurst, radishes, and cucumber

DAY 13

800 calories

BREAKFAST
*(preceded by ten seconds of the
overeater's acupressure):*

1 yogurt
2 thin slices of pumpernickel
2 ounces turkey loaf
Tea or coffee, with milk, if you prefer (sweeten to taste with
artificial sweetener)

IN-BETWEEN MEAL

1 cup clear instant broth

LUNCH
*(preceded by ten seconds of the
overeater's acupressure):*
ASPARAGUS WITH TOMATO SALAD AND HAM

14 ounces asparagus
1 small onion
2 ounces boiled ham (remove all fat)
½ ounce butter
2 small potatoes
3 tomatoes

Trim and, if necessary, skin the asparagus and boil in salted water. Drain it and place it on a heated platter. Pour melted butter over the asparagus and serve it with the ham and the potatoes, boiled in their jackets. Slice the tomatoes and season with chopped onion, salt, and pepper.

IN-BETWEEN MEAL
1 cup consommé or clear instant broth

DINNER
*(preceded by ten seconds of the
overeater's acupressure):*

Mixed salad of Boston lettuce, iceberg lettuce, onions, tomatoes, and radishes with a dressing of low-fat yogurt, a few drops of oil, parsley, dill, and chives
1 thin slice of pumpernickel

DAY 14

800 calories

BREAKFAST
*(preceded by ten seconds of the
overeater's acupressure):*

1 slice whole-wheat bread
2 ounces low-fat cheese
1 tomato
Tea or coffee, with milk, if you prefer (sweeten to taste with artificial sweetener)

IN-BETWEEN MEAL

1 banana (5 ounces)

LUNCH
*(preceded by ten seconds of the
overeater's acupressure):*
HADDOCK IN MUSTARD SAUCE, BOSTON LETTUCE, AND POTATOES

    7 ounces haddock
    2 small potatoes
    ½ ounce butter or margarine
    ½ ounce flour
    1 tsp each prepared mustard, salt, vinegar
    1 cup water or instant broth

Steam haddock. For the sauce, melt the fat over a hot flame
and add the flour, stirring constantly; when flour is light
brown add the liquid slowly, beating it with an eggbeater to
avoid clumps; bring to a boil, then let simmer over a low
flame and season with mustard, vinegar, and salt. Serve with
the boiled potatoes and the salad, prepared with low-fat
yogurt and chives.

IN-BETWEEN MEAL

1 glass tomato juice

DINNER
*(preceded by ten seconds of the
overeater's acupressure):*

1¾ ounces low-fat cottage cheese with chives
   1 slice whole-grain bread
   2 tomatoes

DAY 15

800 calories

BREAKFAST
*(preceded by ten seconds of the
overeater's acupressure):*

1 glass orange juice
2 slices whole-grain bread
2 slices of smoked ham
Tea or coffee, with milk, if you prefer (sweeten to taste with
  artificial sweetener)

IN-BETWEEN MEAL

1 cup low-fat yogurt

LUNCH
*(preceded by ten seconds of the
overeater's acupressure):*
MEAT WITH RICE, VEGETABLES, AND GREEN SALAD

5½ ounces veal, cut in 1-inch cubes
 1 green pepper, diced
1¾ ounces fine peas (frozen)
 2 tbsp rice, uncooked
Water to cover, salt, pepper, curry powder, parsley, sautéd
  chopped onions

Sauté the chopped onions, add the veal and brown, add green
pepper and rice, water to cover and add seasonings, simmer
thirty minutes, add the peas and simmer another five minutes.
Serve a green salad.

IN-BETWEEN MEAL

1 cup clear instant broth

DINNER
*(preceded by ten seconds of the
overeater's acupressure):*

3½ ounces spiced cottage cheese, mixed with a small quantity
of milk, pickles, and cubed tomatoes
2 thin slices of pumpernickel
Radishes

D A Y   1 6

800 calories

BREAKFAST
*(preceded by ten seconds of the
overeater's acupressure):*

2 slices whole-grain bread
1¾ ounces Polish sausage or lean ham
2 tomatoes
Tea or coffee, with milk, if you prefer (sweeten to taste with
artificial sweetener)

IN-BETWEEN MEAL
About 7 ounces of melon (without sugar)

LUNCH
*(preceded by ten seconds of the
overeater's acupressure):*
GRILLED OR BROILED CORNISH GAME HEN

½ small Cornish game hen
1 tsp oil
½ lemon, salt, paprika, pepper, mustard
1¾ ounces salad greens
½ small onion

Rub the chicken with salt and paprika, brush it with oil, and
grill or broil it. Prepare dressing for salad with lemon juice,
salt, pepper, mustard, and minced onion.

IN-BETWEEN MEAL

1 cup consommé or clear instant broth

DINNER
*(preceded by ten seconds of the
overeater's acupressure):*

Carrot salad, made with grated carrots mixed with evaporated
milk, artificial sweetener, and plenty of lemon juice
1 thin slice of pumpernickel

DAY 17

800 calories

BREAKFAST
*(preceded by ten seconds of the
overeater's acupressure):*

1 glass unsweetened grapefruit juice
1 slice graham bread
2 ounces of low-fat cottage cheese
1 tomato
Tea or coffee, with milk, if you prefer (sweeten to taste with
artificial sweetener)

IN-BETWEEN MEAL

1 raw kohlrabi or 2 raw carrots

LUNCH
*(preceded by ten seconds of the
overeater's acupressure):*
POTATO PANCAKES AND APPLESAUCE

2 ready-mix potato pancakes
3 tbsp applesauce for diabetics (if not sweet enough, use artificial sweetener)
1 tsp oil for frying the pancakes

IN-BETWEEN MEAL

7 ounces strawberries (without sugar) or 1 large peach

DINNER
*(preceded by ten seconds of the
overeater's acupressure):*

1 bowl of cucumber/tomato salad with a little oil, vinegar, onion, salt, and pepper
1 thin slice of pumpernickel
1 ounce low-fat soft cheese

DAY 18

800 calories

BREAKFAST
*(preceded by ten seconds of the
overeater's acupressure):*

1 cup yogurt
1 slice of toast
1 tbsp sugar-free jam
Tea or coffee, with milk, if you prefer (sweeten to taste with artificial sweetener)

IN-BETWEEN MEAL

1 apple

LUNCH
*(preceded by ten seconds of the
overeater's acupressure):*
FLOUNDER, ENDIVE SALAD, POTATOES

9 ounces flounder
1 tsp butter
3 small potatoes
Lemon juice, salt, pepper, ½ small onion, parsley, dill

Rub flounder with lemon juice and salt. Broil, grill, or bake it in aluminum foil. Mince the herbs and mix them with the butter; spread them over the flounder. Prepare a dressing for the endives of 3 tbsp low-fat yogurt, onion, salt, and pepper.

IN-BETWEEN MEAL

1 glass skim milk

DINNER
(preceded by ten seconds of the
overeater's acupressure):

2 slices whole-grain bread
4 slices of lean ham
Radishes or green peppers

D A Y   1 9

800 calories

BREAKFAST
(preceded by ten seconds of the
overeater's acupressure):

½ grapefruit
2 slices whole-grain bread
1¾ ounces turkey loaf
Tea or coffee, with milk, if you prefer (sweeten to taste with
   artificial sweetener)

IN-BETWEEN MEAL

1 glass freshly squeezed orange juice

LUNCH
(preceded by ten seconds of the
overeater's acupressure):
PORK CUTLET WITH BRUSSELS SPROUTS

3½ ounces pork cutlet
4½ ounces Brussels sprouts
2 small potatoes
Salt, pepper, paprika

Season cutlet with salt and paprika and grill or broil it on
both sides without fat. Boil sprouts in salted water. Season to
taste with salt and nutmeg.

IN-BETWEEN MEAL

1 glass sauerkraut juice

DINNER
*(preceded by ten seconds of the
overeater's acupressure):*

1 yogurt with strawberries
1 rusk

Mix low-fat yogurt with unsweetened strawberries; if you prefer, add artificial sweetener.

D A Y 2 0

800 calories

BREAKFAST
*(preceded by ten seconds of the
overeater's acupressure):*

1 slice whole-grain bread
3 slices smoked filet of ham
Tea or coffee, with milk, if you prefer (sweeten to taste with artificial sweetener)

IN-BETWEEN MEAL

1 apple (5 ounces)

LUNCH
*(preceded by ten seconds of the
overeater's acupressure):*
SCRAMBLED EGGS WITH MUSHROOMS, ON TOAST

  2 eggs
  1 tbsp evaporated milk
  ½ ounce margarine
  1 slice toast
  2 tomatoes
1¾ ounces canned mushrooms
Salt, pepper, 1 small onion, parsley

Sauté mushrooms in margarine, together with finely chopped onion; season with salt and pepper. Beat the eggs with the evaporated milk; add this to the mushrooms. When the mushrooms are done, place them on warm toast and garnish with parsley. Serve with sliced tomatoes.

IN-BETWEEN MEAL

1 cup consommé or clear instant broth

DINNER
(preceded by ten seconds of the overeater's acupressure):
BREAST OF CHICKEN WITH CHICORY SALAD

3½ ounces cooked breast of chicken
3½ ounces chicory
1¾ ounces orange
1¾ ounces apple
1¾ ounces yogurt
Lemon juice
Artificial sweetener
1 thin slice of pumpernickel

DAY 21

800 calories

BREAKFAST
(preceded by ten seconds of the overeater's acupressure):

1 apricot
6 tbsp cornflakes
5 ounces skim milk
Tea or coffee, with milk, if you prefer (sweeten to taste with artificial sweetener)

IN-BETWEEN MEAL

1 cup clear instant broth

LUNCH
*(preceded by ten seconds of the
overeater's acupressure):*
VEAL CUTLET WITH LEAF SPINACH

3½ ounces veal cutlet
Salt, paprika, nutmeg, garlic salt
  5 ounces spinach
  ½ small onion
  ¼ ounce butter
  2 small potatoes

Season cutlet on both sides with salt and pepper; cook it in a coated pan, or grill it, without fat. Pour boiling water over spinach and drain it. Sauté finely chopped onion in hot butter; add the spinach and sauté about 5 minutes. Season with pepper, nutmeg, and a little garlic salt. Serve with two small boiled potatoes.

IN-BETWEEN MEAL

7 ounces raspberries or strawberries (without sugar)

DINNER
*(preceded by ten seconds of the
overeater's acupressure):*

3½ ounces farmer's cheese, mixed with radishes and 2 tomatoes
  2 thin slices of pumpernickel

REDUCED ENOUGH? DESIRED WEIGHT ACHIEVED?

After the 250–300-calorie starter diet, and the subsequent 800-calorie reducing diet, you should now be pretty close to your ideal weight. If you are not—which may be the case, if you were burdened with a great deal of excess weight —then you should continue, under medical supervision, with the 800-calorie diet that you have become used to by now.

Do so until you are within about 5 percent of your desirable weight (see table on page 14).

You will reach this goal comfortably with the help of acupressure, just as others by the thousands have reached it (even without acupressure and decidedly less comfortably). For instance, in Munich, where I practice, a local newspaper offers year after year a hugely successful "Spring Cure" with slogans like "twenty pounds of fat have to go," along with suitable diet suggestions. Even restaurants follow suit by presenting low-calorie menus recommended by the "Spring Cure," and I am sure that in and around Munich, during those few spring weeks, many tons of surplus body bulk are made to disappear. A most beneficial and laudable result.

The trouble is, it's always the same people who year after year enthusiastically reduce because, in the interval, they have gained back their original overweight. As the "Spring Cure" draws to a close, they are already feverishly anticipating the day when they can at last indulge again. And that is the whole point: Enough willpower can be mustered to reduce. The motives—beauty and health—are strong. But once the goal is reached, all this is forgotten; there is no more reason not to rush back to the old joyous pursuit of food and drink. As I have said, through dieting one can shed the pounds, but not the compulsion.

This is, if you will, the second moment of truth for acupressure: It helps to calm the compulsive-eating center, even when you are basking in the pleasure of being at your ideal weight. What really counts is maintaining this weight—not going through an up-down-up-down cycle, like a yo-yo, as so many do. This is the nub of my acupressure-diet combination: to curb the compulsion to such an extent that even after reduction of weight to a healthy level, there remains no impulse to reacquire what was lost only recently.

For this, apart from acupressure, you again need a diet: a weight-maintenance diet. Its aim is to reliably prevent a return of the lost pounds. It is, therefore, rather narrowly calculated; this leaves a safety margin for restaurant visits, banquets, parties, ice-cream sins, and such-like occurrences. This suggested maintenance diet is slightly below the physiological limit, which is about 12 calories per pound of body weight for a person of nearly ideal weight; this adds up to about 1,800 calories for a man weighing 150 pounds and 1,400 calories for a woman weighing 120 pounds. The diet that you will find on the following pages has about 1,300 calories per day, is low in fat, low in carbohydrates, rich in proteins, and rich in vitamins; it is a diet by which you can live well. If you stay with this 1,300-calorie regimen and feel well, you have made it.

If you should continue to lose weight because you are not taking advantage of the small safety margin for minor sins that has been worked into the diet, then begin to increase the helpings a little when you have reached your ideal weight: steaks one size larger, fish helpings a little bigger, and beverages also somewhat more generous. As long as the scales show no increase in weight, you can continue with this more liberal pattern. You will have succeeded, with acupressure, in establishing a healthy weight, and you will also be able to maintain that weight. It may even happen that after a while you won't need acupressure any longer to curb your urge to eat.

But, all this is for the future. At present, go on your 1,300-calorie maintenance diet. As a rule, you will now need no more protein and vitamin supplements. Medical checkups can become less frequent.

BEVERAGES

As a general rule, even with the 1,300-calorie diet, only drinks very low in calories are allowed: tea or coffee (maximum three cups), with milk, if you wish, but without sugar; mineral water (possibly with a splash of red wine); special low-calorie soft drinks (please watch for listed calorie content); instant broth. Now and then you may have a maximum of one bottle of diet beer or one glass of very dry white wine.

THE WEIGHT-MAINTENANCE DIET: RECIPES

The following recipes are in the nature of general recommendations. They can, of course, be modified according to individual tastes: If you have an aversion toward dairy products, switch to other protein-rich foods; if you do not like one kind of meat, choose another one equally low in fat, or eat fish. Many readers will moan because they believe that in the long run they cannot get along on so few calories. They have not yet experienced how acupressure helps. Other readers will consider the diet recommendations not rigorous enough. They might prefer more stress on natural foods, or a complete nutritional changeover. In their opinion, perhaps, only whole-grain products should be used, or a vegetarian diet should be advocated—or perhaps the opposite—more meat, fish, and eggs, in order to eliminate even more carbohydrates and fat, for a faster weight loss. Please, keep in mind, though, that for thousands of years mankind has subsisted on the main components of protein, carbohydrates, and fat. In the long run, *every* one-sided diet is potentially dangerous. Only fat can be almost totally omitted without any risk.

Therefore, I am repeating once more what I mentioned at the outset: With this book I want to present a practical and risk-free diet method for reducing, which the large army of the "pleasingly plump" can adhere to because it does not require any radical readjustment; because it is not harmful to health, as so many other, one-sided forms of dieting are; and because this diet, combined with acupressure, unfailingly leads to *lasting* success. Of what use is an ever-so-clever health strategy, if aversion quickly makes it unworkable?

Whoever, *over a period of time,* has followed my suggested, easily carried-out plan of nutrition will notice as a welcome side effect that he has become more health-conscious, that his taste in foods has slowly changed—and he will make the happy discovery that high-quality nutrition and enjoyment are not mutually exclusive! And with the loss of the excess "fat pillows" and the resulting gratification, interest in healthful nutrition will increase. Through a reduced, varied food intake, a way to a quality-conscious individual way of eating will be found, without restraints or struggle, adapted to personal taste and way of life. Moreover, the excess pounds will be lost and better health will be gained.

DAY 1

1,300 calories

BREAKFAST
(preceded by five to ten seconds
of the overeater's acupressure):

2 slices light rye bread
3½ ounces low-fat cottage cheese seasoned with caraway seeds and herbs
1¾ ounces boiled ham (fat removed)
Tea or coffee, with milk, if you prefer (sweeten to taste with artificial sweetener)

IN-BETWEEN MEAL
1 glass vegetable juice

LUNCH
(preceded by five to ten seconds
of the overeater's acupressure):
STUFFED PEPPER WITH RICE AND TOMATO SALAD

3½ ounces green pepper
3½ ounces chopped beef
1 onion
Radishes
Salt, pepper, paprika
⅓ ounce margarine
Broth with fat removed
2 ounces cooked rice (3 tbsp)
1 egg
7 ounces tomato salad

Mix the chopped meat with the finely chopped onion and spices; fill the green pepper with the mixture. Melt the margarine, add the pepper and the defatted broth; cook until done.

IN-BETWEEN MEAL

1 apple

DINNER
*(preceded by five to ten seconds
of the overeater's acupressure):*

Fish-filet salad: Mix 3½ ounces cooked haddock with pineapple cubes, finely chopped celery, yogurt-herb dressing, and onion
1 Boston lettuce salad
1 slice wheat bread

DAY 2

1,300 calories

BREAKFAST
*(preceded by five to ten seconds
of the overeater's acupressure):*
SWISS MUESLI

1 ounce Quaker Oats, 1 unpeeled apple
3½ ounce orange
3½ ounce low-fat yogurt
1 tbsp walnuts
Lemon juice, liquid artificial sweetener
Tea or coffee, with milk, if you prefer (sweeten to taste with artificial sweetener)

Peel the orange, wash the apple, and cut both in small slices. Lightly mix all ingredients and season with lemon juice and sweetener.

IN-BETWEEN MEAL

1 glass tomato juice

LUNCH
(preceded by five to ten seconds
of the overeater's acupressure):
BOILED TROUT, PARSLEY POTATOES, GREEN SALAD

9 ounces trout
Salt, lemon juice, 1 bayleaf
3½ ounces potato, parsley
3½ ounces green salad, a few drops of vegetable oil
Lemon juice, chives, dill

Boil water with the lemon juice, the salt, and the bayleaf; place the trout in the boiling liquid, turn the heat down, and simmer for 20 minutes. Serve with melted butter and a lemon slice. For the salad prepare a dressing of oil, lemon juice, salt, chives, and parsley.

IN-BETWEEN MEAL
2 whole-grain rusks or 1 zwieback

DINNER
(preceded by five to ten seconds
of the overeater's acupressure):

2 slices of rye bread
8 slices of smoked ham (3 ounces)

DAY 3

1,300 calories

BREAKFAST
(preceded by five to ten seconds
of the overeater's acupressure):

1 slice mixed-grain bread
1 slice pumpernickel
1¾ ounces turkey loaf
3½ ounces low-fat cottage cheese
1 tomato
Tea or coffee, with milk, if you prefer (sweeten to taste with artificial sweetener)

IN-BETWEEN MEAL

1 glass vegetable broth or defatted broth

LUNCH
*(preceded by five to ten seconds
of the overeater's acupressure):*
BOILED DINNER

4½ ounces lean beef
1 tsp margarine
Salt, pepper, paprika, 1 onion
Defatted broth or water
1¾ ounces turnips, 1¾ ounces carrots, 1¾ ounces cabbage,
   1¾ ounces green beans, 2½ ounces potato, parsley

Cube the beef, melt the margarine, fry the meat on all sides.
Add the chopped onion and sauté. Season the meat. Add
the broth and cook the meat until half done. Place the meat,
vegetables, and potato into an ovenproof casserole with a
cover. Close it tightly and finish cooking the food in the oven.
Sprinkle with chopped parsley before serving.

IN-BETWEEN MEAL

3 small tangerines

DINNER
*(preceded by five to ten seconds
of the overeater's acupressure):*

3½ ounces cold roast veal
1 slice whole-grain bread
1 caraway-seed cracker
1 ounce low-fat soft cheese
Radishes

DAY 4

BREAKFAST
*(preceded by five to ten seconds
of the overeater's acupressure):*

1 slice graham bread
1 rye crisp
1 low-fat yogurt
1 tomato
1 tbsp honey or 1 ounce lean liverwurst or 1¾ ounce turkey
loaf
Tea or coffee, with milk, if you prefer (sweeten to taste with
artificial sweetener)

IN-BETWEEN MEAL

1 grapefruit (unsweetened)

LUNCH
*(preceded by five to ten seconds
of the overeater's acupressure):*
HAM OMELET WITH ASPARAGUS, BOILED POTATO, SALAD

2 eggs
7 ounces asparagus
½ ounce butter
2 slices boiled ham (3 ounces)
Salt, parsley, chives

Beat the eggs with salt and a few drops of water; cook the
omelet in a hot pan, place on a plate, cover with the boiled
asparagus, ham, and melted butter and fold over. Prepare a
salad dressing of yogurt, lemon, and chives.

IN-BETWEEN MEAL

1 glass vegetable juice

DINNER
(preceded by five to ten seconds
of the overeater's acupressure):

1½ ounces low-fat soft cheese
2 slices light rye bread
Radishes and tomatoes

D A Y 5

1,300 calories

BREAKFAST
(preceded by five to ten seconds
of the overeater's acupressure):

2 ounces skim-milk hard cheese
2 slices rye bread
1 apple
Tea or coffee, with milk, if you prefer (sweeten to taste with
artificial sweetener)

IN-BETWEEN MEAL

1 low-fat yogurt

LUNCH
(preceded by five to ten seconds
of the overeater's acupressure):
CHOPPED STEAK, BRUSSELS SPROUTS, AND POTATOES

3½ ounces chopped beef
½ egg, salt, pepper, paprika, 1 small onion
½ ounce margarine
Broth, with the fat removed
7 ounces Brussels sprouts, salt, nutmeg
2 small potatoes

Mix the chopped meat with the half egg, the small chopped
onion, and the seasoning; form a flat patty and fry it on both

sides in a coated pan; add a little defatted broth and finish cooking the meat. Boil the Brussels sprouts in salted water and season with nutmeg.

IN-BETWEEN MEAL

1 cup vegetable broth or 1 beef broth (fat removed)

DINNER
(preceded by five to ten seconds
of the overeater's acupressure):

1 tomato stuffed with cottage cheese and horseradish
1 slice whole-grain bread
1 rye crisp
1½ ounces herring or one ounce lean ham, or 1 ounce tongue, or 2 ounces (4 slices) smoked ham

DAY 6

1,300 calories

BREAKFAST
(preceded by five to ten seconds
of the overeater's acupressure):

1 glass freshly squeezed orange juice
2 slices toast
2 slices boiled ham
1 tbsp honey
Tea or coffee, with milk, if you prefer (sweeten to taste with artificial sweetener)

IN-BETWEEN MEAL

1 cup carrot juice

LUNCH
*(preceded by five to ten seconds
of the overeater's acupressure):*
CHICKEN LEG BAKED IN A BAG, CAULIFLOWER,
AND POTATOES

7-ounce chicken leg (weighed with the bone), salt, paprika
7 ounces cauliflower
Salt, ½ ounce butter
2 small potatoes
Chopped parsley

Wash, dry, and season the chicken leg with salt and paprika.
Place the meat in a Brown-in-Bag and cook according to
instructions on Brown-in-Bag box. Pour the juice from the
bag over the meat. Cook cauliflower in boiling salted water;
serve it with the melted butter and a little nutmeg.

IN-BETWEEN MEAL

Fruit salad: ½ orange, ½ apple, lemon juice, artificial sweetener and 1 tsp rum-flavored extract

DINNER
*(preceded by five to ten seconds
of the overeater's acupressure):*
SHRIMP SALAD

10½ ounces shrimps
Lemon
    1 chopped onion
    1 grated apple
    2 tbsp cooked rice
    2 rye crisps

DAY 7

BREAKFAST
*(preceded by five to ten seconds
of the overeater's acupressure):*

1 glass milk (8 ounces)
1 roll
1 tbsp jam (low-calorie brand)
Tea or coffee, with milk, if you prefer (sweeten to taste with artificial sweetener)

IN-BETWEEN MEAL

1 glass tomato juice

LUNCH
*(preceded by five to ten seconds
of the overeater's acupressure):*
BROILED OR GRILLED SKEWERED BEEF,
TOMATO SALAD, AND RICE

5½ ounces lean beef (filet)
Tomatoes, pickles
  2 small onions
A few drops of vegetable oil
  2 ounces cooked rice (3 tbsp)

Cube the meat, tomatoes, and pickles; slice the onions. Alternating the ingredients, thread the pieces on a skewer; brush with oil. Place the skewer in a preheated broiler and brown on all sides for about 10 minutes; season with salt and pepper. Slice the tomatoes and sprinkle them with salt, pepper, and finely chopped onion.

IN-BETWEEN MEAL

1 low-fat yogurt

DINNER
(preceded by five to ten seconds
of the overeater's acupressure):

2 frankfurters (4½ ounces)
Salad of green peppers and tomatoes, prepared with chopped
onion and herb vinegar
1 slice rye bread
Mustard

D A Y 8

1,300 calories

BREAKFAST
(preceded by five to ten seconds
of the overeater's acupressure):

2 slices whole-grain bread
1 slice boiled ham (fat removed)
1¾ ounces cottage cheese with chives
Tea or coffee, with milk, if you prefer (sweeten to taste with
artificial sweetener)

IN-BETWEEN MEAL

5½ ounces grapes

LUNCH
(preceded by five to ten seconds
of the overeater's acupressure):
BROILED LIVER, SPINACH, AND POTATOES

4½ ounces calf's liver
7 ounces frozen spinach
A few drops of oil
1 small onion
2 small potatoes
Salt, pepper, nutmeg, garlic

Brush the liver on both sides with oil and broil in preheated broiler. After liver is done, season with salt and pepper. Let the spinach thaw slowly over a small flame; add chopped onion, salt, nutmeg, and garlic salt to taste.

IN-BETWEEN MEAL

2 tangerines or 1 apple

DINNER
(preceded by five to ten seconds
of the overeater's acupressure):

3½ ounces beefsteak tartare
  2 slices rye crisp
  1 pickle

D A Y   9

1,300 calories

BREAKFAST
(preceded by five to ten seconds
of the overeater's acupressure):

  1 rye crisp
  1 thin slice wheat bread
3½ ounces chicken roll
  1 ounce low-calorie soft cheese
  2 tomatoes
Tea or coffee, with milk, if you prefer (sweeten to taste with artificial sweetener)

IN-BETWEEN MEAL

1 peach or 1 large orange

LUNCH
*(preceded by five to ten seconds
of the overeater's acupressure):*
STUFFED BEEF ROLL, STRINGBEAN SALAD, POTATOES

4½ ounces thinly sliced beef
  5 ounces stringbeans
Salt, pepper, paprika, mustard
  1 small onion, 1 small pickle
  ½ tomato
A dab of margarine
Defatted broth
  2 small potatoes
  ½ tbsp oil

Season the beef with salt and pepper and spread it with mustard. Distribute the chopped onion, pickle, and tomato over the meat. Roll the meat and tie with thread. Fry the roll on all sides in a coated pan; cover with broth and cook over low heat until done. Marinate the beans in oil, vinegar, salt, pepper, and chopped onion.

IN-BETWEEN MEAL

Vegetable juice

DINNER
*(preceded by five to ten seconds
of the overeater's acupressure):*

2 scrambled eggs
2 tomatoes
1 slice toast

DAY 10

BREAKFAST

*(preceded by five to ten seconds
of the overeater's acupressure):*

2 slices whole-grain bread
1 slice of lean sausage
1¾ ounces soft cheese
Tea or coffee, with milk, if you prefer (sweeten to taste with
   artificial sweetener)

IN-BETWEEN MEAL

1 apple

LUNCH

*(preceded by five to ten seconds
of the overeater's acupressure):*
PORK FILET, TOMATO SALAD, AND MUSHROOM RICE

5 ounces pork filet
Salt, pepper, onion
3 small tomatoes
Radishes

Fry the filet without fat and season it with salt and pepper.
Sauté 2 tbsp rice (uncooked) in ½ tsp oil with ½ onion for
about 12 minutes; add mushrooms and parsley and cook until
done.

IN-BETWEEN MEAL

1 low-fat yogurt

DINNER
*(preceded by five to ten seconds
of the overeater's acupressure):*

Mixed salad of Boston lettuce, tangerine slices, cucumber, tomato, mushrooms, a little broiled, cubed chicken, with a dressing of low-fat yogurt, lemon juice, salt, pepper, and onion powder. Garnish with a little watercress.

1 slice rye bread

DAY 11

1,300 calories

BREAKFAST
*(preceded by five to ten seconds
of the overeater's acupressure):*

2 apricots or a good-sized apple
1 slice toast
3½ ounces cocktail sausages or 3 ounces cold roast turkey
1 tomato
Tea or coffee, with milk, if you prefer (sweeten to taste with artificial sweetener)

IN-BETWEEN MEAL

3½ ounces fresh plums or an orange

LUNCH
*(preceded by five to ten seconds
of the overeater's acupressure):*
STEAMED CODFISH ON A BED OF LEEKS, WITH RICE

9 ounces codfish filet
11 ounces leeks
Salt, pepper, parsley, lemon juice
⅓ ounce margarine
2 tbsp cooked rice

Wash the leeks and cut in pieces. Melt the margarine in a casserole and sauté the vegetable in it, until only half done. Cut the fish into cubes, sprinkle it with lemon juice, and place it on top of the vegetables. Salt it and cook it until it's done. Garnish with chopped parsley.

IN-BETWEEN MEAL

8 ounces chicken broth (defatted)

DINNER
(preceded by five to ten seconds
of the overeater's acupressure):

3½ ounces smoked boiled beef tongue cut in cubes and seasoned with chopped pickle, tomato sauce, and lemon.
1 slice whole-grain bread

D AY 1 2

1,300 calories

BREAKFAST
(preceded by five to ten seconds
of the overeater's acupressure):

1 slice rye crisp
3½ ounces low-fat cottage cheese
1 tomato
Tea or coffee, with milk, if you prefer (sweeten to taste with artificial sweetener)

IN-BETWEEN MEAL

9 ounces melon (without sugar)

LUNCH
*(preceded by five to ten seconds
of the overeater's acupressure):*

HUNGARIAN GOULASH, TOMATO SALAD, AND POTATOES

5½ ounces beef
½ ounce margarine
2 small onions
Beef broth (defatted)
Salt, pepper, paprika
2 small boiled potatoes

Fry the cubed beef on all sides in the hot margarine; add
chopped onions, and cover with hot broth. Cook at medium
heat. Season the tomato salad with salt, pepper, and chopped
onion.

IN-BETWEEN MEAL

1 grapefruit (11 ounces)

DINNER
*(preceded by five to ten seconds
of the overeater's acupressure):*

1 triangle low-fat soft cheese (a little over 2 ounces)
¾ ounce lean liverwurst
1 slice whole-grain bread, one slice white bread
Radishes

DAY 13

1,300 calories

BREAKFAST
*(preceded by five to ten seconds
of the overeater's acupressure):*

1 slice whole-grain bread or one roll
1 tbsp jam (low-calorie)
1 slice rye crisp
1 slice boiled ham (fat removed)
Tea or coffee, with milk, if you prefer (sweeten to taste with
artificial sweetener)

IN-BETWEEN MEAL

1 cup low-fat yogurt

LUNCH
*(preceded by five to ten seconds
of the overeater's acupressure):*
SCRAMBLED EGGS WITH MUSHROOMS, ACCOMPANIED BY
BOSTON LETTUCE OR ENDIVE SALAD

2 eggs
7 ounces mushrooms
1 small onion
½ ounce margarine
Salt, pepper, parsley
2 small boiled potatoes

Sauté mushrooms in the margarine, together with finely chopped onion. Season with salt and pepper; garnish with chopped parsley; serve with potatoes and salad.

IN-BETWEEN MEAL

1 cup chicken broth (defatted)

DINNER
*(preceded by five to ten seconds
of the overeater's acupressure):*
MIXED COLD-CUTS PLATTER

1¾ ounces smoked salmon
1 ounce cold roast turkey
1 ounce liverwurst
1 slice rye bread, 1 slice pumpernickel
Radishes and tomatoes

DAY 14

1,300 calories

BREAKFAST
*(preceded by five to ten seconds
of the overeater's acupressure):*
SWISS MUESLI

1 ounce Quaker Oats
1 unpeeled apple
3½ ounces orange
3½ ounces low-fat yogurt
1 tbsp chopped walnuts
Lemon juice, liquid artificial sweetener
Tea or coffee, with milk, if you prefer (sweeten to taste with
   artificial sweetener)

Preparation: see Day 2 of 1,300-calorie diet.

IN-BETWEEN MEAL

1 slice rye crisp with ½ ounce lean liverwurst

LUNCH
*(preceded by five to ten seconds
of the overeater's acupressure):*
CHICKEN CASSEROLE

7 ounces chicken breast
3½ ounces carrots
2 ounces mushrooms
3½ ounces cauliflower
Chicken broth (defatted)
2 tbsp cooked rice
Parsley
2 ounces green peas

Place all ingredients in the casserole together with some defatted broth and spices; cook until done.

IN-BETWEEN MEAL

1 pear

DINNER
*(preceded by five to ten seconds
of the overeater's acupressure):*
CHEESE PLATTER

1 slice graham bread, 1 slice rye crisp
2 ounces Camembert (low-fat)
3 tbsp low-fat cottage cheese with herbs
1 tomato

DAY 15

1,300 calories

BREAKFAST
*(preceded by five to ten seconds
of the overeater's acupressure):*

2 thin slices sesame-seed bread
1 slice pumpernickel
1¾ ounces chicken roll
1 ounce low-fat soft cheese
1 tomato
Tea or coffee, with milk, if you prefer (sweeten to taste with artificial sweetener)

IN-BETWEEN MEAL

1 orange

LUNCH
*(preceded by five to ten seconds
of the overeater's acupressure):*
FRANKFURTERS, SAUERKRAUT SALAD, AND BOILED POTATOES

7 ounces raw sauerkraut
3½ ounces grated apple
2 frankfurters (4½ ounces)
2 small potatoes

Mix the sauerkraut with grated apple. Heat frankfurters for 2–3 minutes in boiling water. Serve with mustard.

IN-BETWEEN MEAL

1 cup low-fat yogurt

DINNER
(preceded by five to ten seconds of the overeater's acupressure):
FLORIDA TOAST

1 slice toast
2 ounces pineapple
1½ ounces boiled ham
1 ounce low-fat cheese
1 tomato

Toast the bread, cover with ham and pineapple and the cheese; place under broiler.

DAY 16

1,300 calories

BREAKFAST
(preceded by five to ten seconds of the overeater's acupressure):

1 slice whole-grain bread
1 slice rye crisp
3½ ounces low-fat cottage cheese spiced with pickle and tomato
1 tbsp honey
Tea or coffee, with milk, if you prefer (sweeten to taste with artificial sweetener)

IN-BETWEEN MEAL

3 small tangerines or half a melon (small)

LUNCH
*(preceded by five to ten seconds
of the overeater's acupressure):*
VEAL FRICASSEE AND SALAD

7 ounces veal
3½ ounces asparagus
2 tbsp sliced mushrooms
1 tbsp flour
1 egg yolk
Lemon
1 pat of butter

Bind the broth from the boiled meat and vegetables with the flour and yolk, spice with lemon juice, and enrich with the butter. Place the meat, cubed, into the sauce. Serve with 3 tbsp cooked rice and the salad. Prepare salad dressing with 3 tbsp low-fat yogurt, dill, and salt.

IN-BETWEEN MEAL
8-ounce glass of cranberry cocktail (diet brand)

DINNER
*(preceded by five to ten seconds
of the overeater's acupressure):*
HADDOCK IN A BONNET

Place the boiled haddock in a buttered, portion-size fireproof dish; cover with sautéd onion cubes, mustard, parsley, and lemon juice; leave for 5 minutes in a hot oven. Cover with stiffly beaten egg white into which the lightly beaten yolk has been carefully folded, and salt and lemon juice added. Return to oven for another 15 minutes. Serve with 1 potato or 3 tbsp cooked rice, and cucumber salad.

DAY 17

BREAKFAST
*(preceded by five to ten seconds
of the overeater's acupressure):*

1 slice rye bread
1 slice pumpernickel
¾ ounce lean liverwurst
1 egg
1 tomato
Tea or coffee, with milk, if you prefer (sweeten to taste with
artificial sweetener)

IN-BETWEEN MEAL

1 orange

LUNCH
*(preceded by five to ten seconds
of the overeater's acupressure):*

FILET MIGNON WITH MUSHROOMS, TOMATO SALAD,
AND POTATOES

7 ounces filet mignon
3½ ounces mushrooms
½ ounce margarine
2 small potatoes (3½ ounces)
1 small onion
Salt, pepper, 1 tsp oil

Brush filet on both sides with oil; season and broil on both
sides. Sauté chopped onion until glazed; add the mushrooms;
season, and place on the broiled filet. Quarter tomato and
season with onion, salt, and pepper.

IN-BETWEEN MEAL

1 banana or 10 ounces melon slices

DINNER
*(preceded by five to ten seconds
of the overeater's acupressure):*

1 triangle packaged low-fat soft cheese
1 slice whole-grain bread
1 small bunch radishes

D A Y   1 8

1,300 calories

BREAKFAST
*(preceded by five to ten seconds
of the overeater's acupressure):*

1 slice whole-grain bread
2 slices rye crisp
1 tbsp jam (sugar-free)
2 ounces low-fat cottage cheese
1 tomato
Tea or coffee, with milk, if you prefer (sweeten to taste with
artificial sweetener)

IN-BETWEEN MEAL

1 apple

LUNCH
*(preceded by five to ten seconds
of the overeater's acupressure):*

SLICED KIDNEY, GREEN SALAD, POTATOES IN THEIR JACKETS

5½ ounces calf or pork kidney
  1 tsp oil, salt, pepper, mustard, 1 tsp flour
  1 medium potato
  2 tbsp buttermilk
  1 small Boston lettuce
lemon juice, celery salt, herbs

Free the kidney of tendons, skin, and fat; soak it in water; slice
it and fry it in oil. Season with salt and pepper and sprinkle
with the flour. Add a little water to make a sauce; add butter-

milk and mustard to taste. Serve with the potatoes and the salad in a dressing of lemon juice, celery salt, and fresh herbs.

IN-BETWEEN MEAL

1 cup tea or broth (defatted)

DINNER
*(preceded by five to ten seconds
of the overeater's acupressure):*

Chicken salad: 7-ounce chicken leg. Remove the bone, cube, and mix with 3½ ounces cooked asparagus, ½ tangerine, 1 tbsp mayonnaise, a little sharp mustard, 2 tbsp low-fat yogurt, 1 tbsp peas, salt, pepper, and lemon juice.
1 slice rye crisp

D A Y   1 9

1,300 calories

BREAKFAST
*(preceded by five to ten seconds
of the overeater's acupressure):*

2 slices rye crisp
1 slice whole-grain bread
2 slices smoked ham
1 tbsp honey
Tea or coffee, with milk, if you prefer (sweeten to taste with artificial sweetener)

IN-BETWEEN MEAL

1 cup yogurt

LUNCH
*(preceded by five to ten seconds
of the overeater's acupressure):*
MEATBALLS OF VEAL ON PEACH HALVES

Mix 4½ ounces of chopped veal, 1 tbsp evaporated milk, 1 egg, 1 chopped, sautéd onion, parsley, salt, nutmeg, breadcrumbs, and shape into small balls; cook them in broth and place into three warmed peach halves. Serve with 3 tbsp cooked saffron rice.

IN-BETWEEN MEAL

Small fruit salad, made of 1 banana, ½ orange, 3½ ounces apple, juice of 1 lemon, and artificial sweetener.

DINNER
*(preceded by five to ten seconds
of the overeater's acupressure):*
TOMATO EGGS

3 tomatoes
2 eggs
4 tbsp water
Salt, pepper
1 slice rye crisp

Slice the tomatoes thin, place them in a coated pan and fry them briefly. Then add the other ingredients, beaten together, and permit to set, with care.

D A Y 2 0

1,300 calories

BREAKFAST
*(preceded by five to ten seconds
of the overeater's acupressure):*

1 soft-boiled egg
2 slices white bread
½ ounce lean liverwurst
1 tomato
Tea or coffee, with milk, if you prefer (sweeten to taste with artificial sweetener)

IN-BETWEEN MEAL

3½ ounces cherries or 3½ ounces fresh plums

LUNCH
*(preceded by five to ten seconds
of the overeater's acupressure):*
SALMON BAKED IN FOIL, GREEN SALAD, AND POTATOES

7 ounces salmon filet
Salt, lemon juice, herbs
1 small onion
3 small potatoes (5½ ounces)
1 tsp butter

Sprinkle the fish filet with lemon juice and place it on a piece of aluminum foil; cover the fish with the herbs and minced onion. Close the foil tightly and cook the fish in the preheated oven or broiler for 20 minutes. Prepare a mixed green salad with a dressing of 1 teaspoon oil, vinegar, onion, salt, and pepper.

IN-BETWEEN MEAL

1 cup low-fat yogurt with raspberries or strawberries (unsweetened)

DINNER
*(preceded by five to ten seconds
of the overeater's acupressure):*

3 slices of roast beef (3½ ounces)
1 slice rye bread
3½ ounces asparagus

DAY 21

1,300 calories

BREAKFAST
(preceded by five to ten seconds
of the overeater's acupressure):

1 slice graham bread
1 slice toast
1 low-fat yogurt mixed with 3½ ounces strawberries and a little liquid artificial sweetener
1¾ ounces ham (fat removed)
Tea or coffee, with milk, if you prefer (sweeten to taste with artificial sweetener)

IN-BETWEEN MEAL

1 glass tomato juice

LUNCH
(preceded by five to ten seconds
of the overeater's acupressure):
LEG OF VENISON WITH APPLE SALAD

Roast 7 ounces of venison with juniper berries, onion, soup greens, and herbs; serve with 5 tbsp mashed potatoes. For roasting the meat, use a dab of margarine. To prepare the apple salad, mix 3½ ounces of cubed apple with plenty of lemon juice and a little artificial sweetener.

IN-BETWEEN MEAL

8 ounces buttermilk

DINNER
(preceded by five to ten seconds
of the overeater's acupressure):

7 ounces boiled calf's tongue, cubed and mixed with tomato sauce, sliced pickle, and lemon juice. Serve with 3 tbsp rice cooked in bouillion.

ACUPRESSURE—AS THE PATIENTS SEE IT

PATIENT ANTHONY SMITH
(All names have been changed.)

He is forty-four years old, five feet seven inches tall, and weighed 216 pounds. He has a supervisory desk job with the telephone company. His main problem was that he could hardly look at anything edible without immediately wanting it. He characterized himself as "a habitual glutton."

Mr. Smith tried several reducing methods to rid himself of the unhealthy ballast which, he felt, he carried around because of his professional advancement. As he tells it: "I started out laying cables with a construction crew that exchanged cables, sometimes underground, sometimes on telephone poles. That was strenuous labor, and when I was twenty years old I could eat as much meat and drink as many glasses of beer as I pleased, and there wasn't an ounce of fat on my body."

After a time, when he did not plant telephone poles any longer, but controlled switches from an office, the overweight began to accumulate. And in spite of his exaggerated urge to eat, he submitted to an egg cure. That works like this: in the morning three hard-boiled eggs, at noon three hard-boiled eggs and a salad, in the evening three hard-boiled eggs. Or, ten hard-boiled eggs distributed over the day, and a juicy steak at noon.

Such methods are usually recommended as weekend shockers, but Mr. Smith was more thorough; he ate only eggs until he couldn't look at them any longer, and lost a lot of pounds. However, after the cure, noodles and sizzling steaks had by no means lost their attraction for Mr. Smith. Shortly after the egg orgy, he had his old overweight problem once again.

Fall had come, and Mr. Smith tried grape juice—for a

whole week, only three pints of freshly pressed grape juice every day, with nothing else. That also was quite effective, but it cannot be kept up for any length of time.

Other attempts followed, always with the same result: ten, fourteen, sometimes even eighteen pounds were lost and then, either quickly or more slowly, the old weight was regained. This went on until I recommended to him, a few months ago, the acupressure-diet combination. Now Mr. Smith is lighter by thirty pounds; he continues to live trouble-free on a 1,300-calorie diet that allows him an ongoing gradual weight loss. Mr. Smith comments: "I decided to get back to a normal weight because I did not want to be excluded any longer from the joys of life. Thanks to acupressure, there are no indications whatsoever that I might relapse into compulsive eating."

PATIENT EVE HANSEN

Looking at her today, you wouldn't be able to guess what a butterball she was only a short time ago. The thirty-six-year-old, dark-haired, pretty woman, who is only five feet tall, weighed in at 174 pounds. She had started to put on weight by overeating at about age thirty—not because of some unhappiness, but for just the opposite reason. Her husband's business, where she holds an executive position, flourished, the number of invitations of a business and social nature increased, and with them grew Mrs. Hansen's girth.

Mrs. Hansen commented: "One of the problems in our society is the fact that an invitation to a meal is looked upon as a sort of reward. In addition it is a social obligation. It is easy to put on weight when one doesn't feel like saying 'no' to a host or hostess."

In her own judgment, she is a typical "appetite eater"; hunger doesn't enter the picture. So, as time went by, she acquired a barrel shape that her husband, understandably enough, didn't consider particularly attractive; it also became a burden to her in another way—she became short of breath and less mobile.

As she was an "appetite eater," she logically tried to curb her rush to the heaping platter by an appetite depressant. The drug had a negative effect on her and, just in time, symptoms of excessive pressure building in her lungs were detected. (The appetite depressant with this life-endangering side effect was soon afterward withdrawn from the market.)

Of course, not all appetite depressants are dangerous; but as with most medications meant to replace natural behavior, here too the effectiveness is quickly reduced with habitual use, ever larger doses are needed (as in the case of sleeping pills), and from a certain quantity on, even rather harmless drugs may cause damaging and, most of all, unpredictable side effects.

Since Mrs. H. has learned to use acupressure, she can suppress her appetite. She eats now only when she is really hungry and is losing weight steadily. At present, she weighs only 124 pounds, she wears clothes two sizes smaller than previously, her breathing and mobility are restored, and there is no doubt that Mrs. Hansen will reach her goal—110 pounds—and later will be able to maintain this healthy weight.

PATIENT ANN HUNTER

Miss Hunter was one of the first patients on whom the acupressure-diet combination was tried. She is twenty-nine years old; as head of a civil service department, she is subject to considerable strain at her job. In spite of this, until she was twenty-seven years old, her weight was a healthy 110 pounds at a height of five feet two inches. Then, after simultaneous emotional and physical crises—a longstanding relationship broke up and, because of adverse effects, her contraceptive pills had to be discontinued—Miss Hunter gained 22 pounds within a year.

During that time, especially in the evenings and on week-ends, she suffered frequently from depression, which she tried to combat by eating; by her own admission, she was able to eat as much as she wanted to, without ever feeling sick—and she liked to eat everything.

For a year, Miss Hunter tried to regain her previous weight through a variety of starvation diets, but without lasting success. It was characteristic of her to place great hope in one of the startling and famous fad diets, which lets you eat unlimited quantities of fats and proteins while eliminating all carbohydrates. She lost weight, but nevertheless soon stopped; the diet somehow did not seem wholesome. And not without reason! Like all one-sided diets, this wonder diet, too, has its pitfalls; you simply cannot live on fat for any length of time with impunity. The fat content of the blood is danger-ously raised and increases the risk of hardening of the arteries and heart infarct. Another damaging effect of that diet is ketosis. Because of these consequences of the diet, the author is being severely criticized by his medical colleagues.

Back to Miss Hunter. She stopped the diet, despite the little effort it required, and tried others. She even lost some weight, but neither lastingly nor in the right places; to her annoyance, the weight loss was apparent above her waistline and not on her hips and thighs, where the disfiguring fat had mainly settled.

Miss Hunter then learned how to use acupressure. It was possible to relieve her depressed mood by eliminating some other problems in consultation with her doctor. Result: Miss Hunter has her former weight of 110 pounds back; her figure, too, has regained its proper shape; and she does not go in for weekend eating anymore.

Her comment: "It was great to lose weight with the help of acupressure, but I found out that in addition to the physi-cal change, a new psychological attitude is necessary. A friend of mine, as I became slimmer, suddenly lost all interest in me—perhaps she was afraid that I had again become interesting to men. Yes, I even had problems with men friends who became envious and suspicious."

PATIENT FRANK STANTON

This case is a little out of the ordinary because of the youth of the patient, the nineteen-year-old Frank Stanton. He is very tall—six feet four inches. But even for that height, 220 pounds are definitely too many, especially for a man of Mr. Stanton's fine-boned frame. Thirty pounds less would be about right, and that was Mr. Stanton's weight when he was sixteen years old and already just as tall.

Strangely enough, it was precisely the sport that he took up at that time that caused his gradual weight gain. Frank Stanton went in for sailing, not just for pleasure, but competitively. Whoever is familiar with regatta sailing knows the rough conditions, the tricks, the protests and so forth, and knows how much stress is caused by this competitive sport. This racing stress noticeably increased Mr. Stanton's appetite. He just ate and ate, without giving it a thought, as young people will. What nineteen-year-old would worry about his weight?—especially one so tall. And many a sailor not only loves water under his keel, but also liquor in his glass. So, Frank raised the elbow together with his sailing partners, and raised it again and all this drinking contributed to turning the tall, slender youth into a 220-pound man. Once he had reached the 220-pound mark, he began to realize that this was simply too much. He started to take appetite depressants, but achieved only a minor weight reduction that, moreover, did not last. For the next step, he had a so-called computer diet set up for himself. He reports: "What I was supposed to eat, I did not like—it was really awful stuff. But I thought, perhaps that's how it has to be, and stuck to the diet. Only, after I ate the stuff, I was still ravenously hungry, and I just can't take being hungry all the time." So he ate other things in addition, and did not lose weight.

From a friend, he heard of the acupressure-diet combination. It brought quick results and Frank reached his goal, a thirty-pound loss, in a surprisingly short time.

PATIENT GRACE TASKER

Grace Tasker is an exceptionally good-looking and well-groomed thirty-five-year-old woman. At five feet six inches she weighed 150 pounds. This was not really a serious overweight problem, but she wanted to lose at least fifteen pounds, for professional reasons. She is a cosmetician, has to travel, and has to display a perfect figure; and this perfect appearance, as she well knows, requires in her case a weight of around 130 pounds.

She kept that weight, and the matching good figure, until a change in jobs that brought with it some aggravations and altered the rhythm of her life in a way that left her with more free time on her hands—and with more time for eating. Sometimes she ate out of sheer boredom. Attempts to lose weight, first with a potato diet, then with appetite depressants, finally through self-hypnosis, were unsuccessful.

Miss Tasker described the, for her crucial, effect of acupressure: "It's strange how I can restrain myself now, something I was not capable of before. I now really eat only what I need. To be slim is a status symbol today. The jet-setters and the rich are all slim (in contrast to the past, when they were fat) and for this reason everyone tries to emulate them." She is now only four pounds away from her dream weight and her job-required dream figure.

PATIENT MATILDA EMORY

Matilda Emory, a fifty-seven-year-old married woman with one son, works full-time as a computer programmer. At five feet five inches, she weighed in at 184 pounds—much too fat. This did not bother her. The excess pounds had slowly accumulated over the years; she had become accustomed to them and had no incentive whatsoever to reduce.

The incentive was provided by her family physician. She suffered from very painful arthritis of both knee joints and constantly requested pain-killing medication from this doctor; he finally refused her, with the appropriate explanation that first the ailing knees would have to be relieved of the excess burden they constantly had to support. Her doctor suggested a zero-diet in a hospital. Because of a recent operation, she had to stay several weeks in a hospital where, through the enforced bed rest, she had developed thrombosis in both legs. This extremely disagreeable experience caused her to reject any hospital stay not absolutely necessary, and she categorically refused. But she did realize that she had to reduce radically.

She tried, tenaciously, four different diets: a potato diet, the Hollywood diet, a banana diet, an egg diet. Mrs. Emory sums up her experience in the concise language of her profession: "I more or less weighed more or less." She was only too willing to give acupressure a try. The outcome proved her right. Mrs. Emory is now twenty pounds lighter—not nearly enough—but the arthritis pain in her now much-less-burdened knee joints has eased up to the point where most of the time it is tolerable without medication. Mrs. Emory is in the process of slowly losing another twenty pounds; she assures me that this will be "not at all difficult."

EXERCISE, EXERCISE, EXERCISE!

Aside from the urge to overeat, lack of exercise is one of the main causes of the common tendency to become obese. Most modern men and women only walk from their bed to the bathroom, then to the breakfast table, where they sit, then to the garage or to the bus, only a few steps away; there they sit again, and after another few steps to their place of work, they sit once more. This is true not only of those who are office workers, but also of the crane operator in his cab, the trucker, the man who directs the red-hot steel sheets through the rolling mill—they all earn their living while sitting down. After working hours and some few intermediary movements, they conclude their day by sitting in front of the television set.

This increasing lack of exercise—the fat person finds it difficult to move, becomes sluggish, moves even less, gets fatter still—has to be counteracted, and not only for the purpose of burning calories. Man is not built for a sedentary, inactive life; he *has* to move if he wants to stay healthy. Muscles that are not exercised become slack and finally waste away; joints that are not used may even gradually stiffen.

How much the human structure is geared to movement can be seen in the main supply system of this nearly perfect machine—the circulatory system—the workings of which also depend on movement. Although fresh blood is sent through the arteries to its destination by means of a pressure pump, the heart, the return of the blood through the veins is partly effected by a squeezing of the veins caused by the tensing and relaxing of the surrounding muscles. There are valves at short intervals in the veins, which allows only a one-way flow of the blood—toward the heart. When the veins are squeezed together by the muscular system, the blood is pushed toward the heart; it cannot flow backward. With lack of exercise, the veins become lax, the valves do not properly close any longer, and the veins quickly become diseased—varicose veins, for instance, are an affliction almost exclusively of fat or physically lazy people.

THE IDLE WHEEL RUSTS

Sufficient exercise is a must also, and especially, during an acupressure-diet cure. Exercise means increased energy expenditure: that is, reduction of the body's fat reserves.

It is, no doubt, discouraging to figure out that twenty-five hours of walking are necessary to lose one single pound. Under these circumstances it seems rather ridiculous to advise overweight executives to leave their chauffeured limousine two blocks from their destination and walk that short distance; that doesn't amount to very much. It would be a different proposition if the overweight captain of industry were asked to climb the stairs up to the twelfth-floor executive suite instead of taking the elevator. Hoisting 175 pounds up 120 feet is no mean task; if done regularly and at a good clip, this would rid a person of half a pound per week.

Nevertheless, I would not recommend rapid and extensive stair-climbing to an untrained overweight person for a setting-up exercise, at least not for a starter. The energy expenditure there is so high and the sudden overload for heart and circulation so violent that complications could easily arise. Even someone climbing very leisurely to the twelfth floor will arrive there with wobbly knees, muscle pains, and an accelerated pulse, out of breath and with perspiration on his forehead.

Nevertheless, people with offices on high floors should definitely use the stairs as a training ground, but without overdoing it. As a beginning, walk up only about three flights, slowly, and travel the rest of the way by elevator; gradually the speed can be increased until the three flights can be rushed up two steps at a time, without a disagreeable rise in breathing rate and pulse rate. Once this is achieved, two more flights can be added, by climbing them at first slowly, then faster, and so forth.

Don't get overly ambitious. Don't overexert yourself. Since the fitness movement started, people who have overdone it have crowded into doctors' offices; with bones, tendons, ligaments, and joints that for years were hardly used, one cannot run and jump like a seventeen-year-old. If one attempts it nevertheless, then something breaks, tears, or strains, especially when, in addition, the "old bones" carry much more weight than they rightly should. The frequently already-fat-clogged heart suddenly has to perform extra-heavy labor; many who strenuously worked at regaining a youthful shape have succumbed to a heart attack along the jogging trail or at the exercise machine.

The first question, then, before beginning to use up extra energy and break down fat through vigorous exercise, is:

WHAT ARE MY LIMITS?

First of all: If you want to start an effective energy-expenditure training program you should have a thorough medical checkup, and tell your doctor what you are planning to do.

Then, there is a useful rule of thumb for gauging the advisable limit of exertion: The pulse rate, during exertion, should not exceed 180-minus-your-age per minute; that is about 130 beats for a man of fifty.

If the effort is not great—causing little rise in pulse rate— the conditioning effect for all muscles, including the heart muscle, is not yet optimal; on the other hand, exceeding the correct pulse rate can only lead to early exhaustion and over-burdening of the heart. To pace yourself according to the optimal pulse rate, you have to check your pulse once in a while during training, at your wrist or at the carotid artery, for a period of fifteen seconds, then multiply the number by four. Therefore, you have to carry a watch when you exercise. After a while you will know your optimal rate, even without constant checking. Observe this rule: When your breath gets short and the pulse beat becomes disagreeably noticeable, it is time for a rest; that is, continue slowly until pulse and breathing have quieted down (pulse down to 100), then increase your effort once more. Don't stop before you are perspiring lightly. This holds true for all types of exercise that involve considerable energy expenditure.

1) HIKING, RUNNING

Regrettably, these forms of exercise are within the reach of only those with the necessary time and opportunity, yet they are among the best means for reconditioning the body. Very

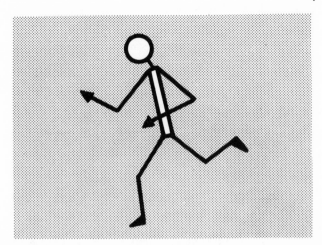

heavy people should not start right away with lively jogging that the tendons, ligaments, and joints might resent, but should, instead, begin with steady walks at about three and a half miles per hour. This does not greatly affect the energy balance (up to 350 calories per hour), but does crank up the body.

Running, long-distance running, and jogging use up more calories (up to 500 per hour). Be sure to wear suitable foot-wear. If at all possible, avoid running on asphalt or other hard surfaces; preferably, use a solid grassy surface or a path in the woods. Jog at even pace, not in spurts, and take needed rests. It's best to run over a level stretch, not uphill (certainly not at the beginning), or the strain might become too great.

2) SWIMMING

Also, a question of opportunity, and also very beneficial, since heart, lungs, and all the muscles are equally involved. It is particularly suitable for very heavy people since tendons, ligaments, and joints are not burdened. The energy expenditure, depending on the speed of the swimmer, is rather higher than with running (up to 600 calories per hour). Of course,

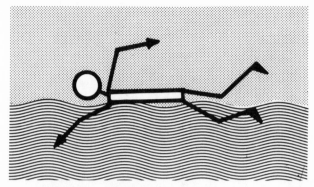

you cannot leisurely paddle along, in the way one often sees people in pools endlessly swimming back and forth at a snail's pace, marveling at their own achievement.

Certainly, that too is good and healthy, but the resulting energy expenditure is not much greater than during a leisurely stroll (about 110 calories an hour). If you swim to speed up your reducing, you will have to do a little more—swim as fast as you possibly can. If you find you are already out of breath after the first lap, then take a rest before starting on the next one. In any case, the body has to become adjusted to the unfamiliar exertion. If you continue to swim regularly, after a few weeks you will be able to do several laps at a good speed and without stopping to rest; this will help with the weight and—a special advantage of swimming—with your figure.

3) BICYCLE RIDING

This permits you to spend quite a bit of energy in a comparatively pleasant fashion (up to about 400 to 500 calories per hour). At the outset don't pedal uphill, wheezing and puffing (the exertion is too great). Bicycling is as well suited as swimming to the severely overweight. Pace yourself carefully, the same as with running, and increase the effort gradually.

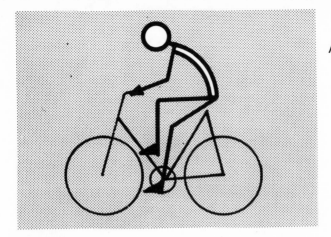

4) DANCING

This is not a recommendation to go dancing every night—that would inevitably lead to taking forbidden drinks. But one can also dance at home, and lively dances like the rhumba, samba, waltz, and hustle generate a lot of movement; the energy expenditure matches that of running.

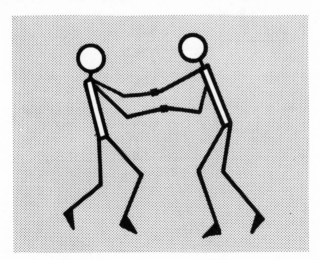

5) EXERCISES

Some people may lack the time, others the opportunity, for bicycling, running, or swimming. But everybody has the room and the ten minutes before breakfast to do some exercises.

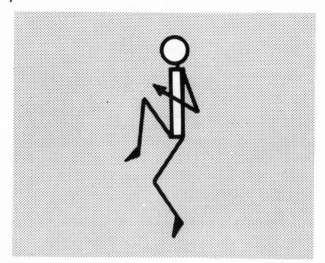

a) *Running in place.* Run barefoot, on a carpeted floor. Lift the knees as high as possible, almost up to your chest. A program of running like the one done outdoors; this means you should stay within the prescribed pulse range during exertion.

b) *Rope jumping.* Not suited for very heavy people (it over-

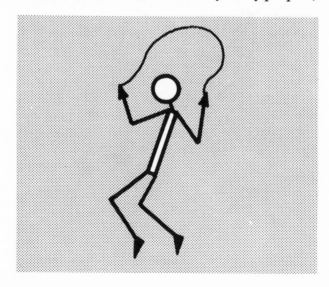

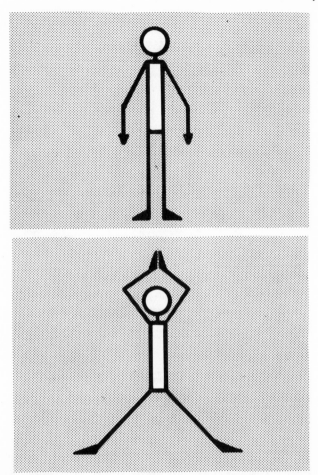

taxes the joints), but good for the moderately overweight. It gives the body a good shaking-up.

c) *Jumping jack.* Stand erect, feet together, arms hanging down loosely. Jump up, and come down with slightly spread legs while at the same time swinging your stretched arms upward until your hands meet above your head. Immediately return to starting position and repeat the jumps in quick succession, in imitation of a jumping jack.

d) *Knee bends.* If you are greatly overweight, do not do

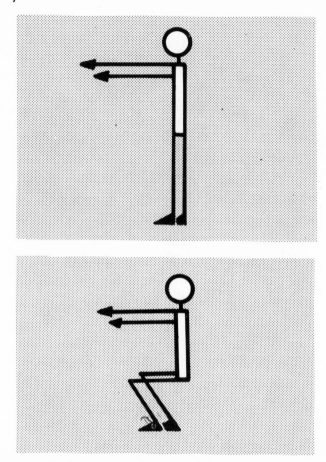

knee bends too quickly or too many times. Rhythmically rise and bend, with arms stretched out at shoulder level.

All the above exercises use up considerable energy; if you spend ten minutes in the morning doing them, and afterward, slightly perspiring, take your bath, you will have done a lot toward keeping yourself nimble and reducing your weight. Going only by the numbers, the ounces of fat you lose during morning exercises may not add up to a whole lot; the end effect, though, in combination with diet and acupressure, will be much greater.

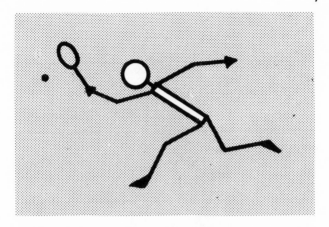

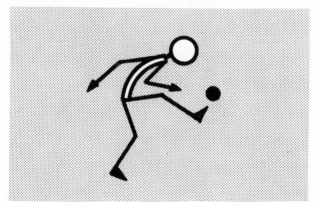

Our principle: the exercise you prefer for the burning of calories is the best for you; otherwise you might not go beyond the good intention! Most overweight people prefer to combine the burning of calories with sports like tennis, soccer, or a similar sweat-inducing exercise. It is important, though, to quench the resulting thirst with low-calorie drinks only.

EXERCISES AIMED AT CRITICAL POINTS— EXERCISES THAT YOU WILL ENJOY!

"I exercise for beauty," says the movie idol Farrah Fawcett-Majors, who starts her day with seven minutes of exercise. Imi-

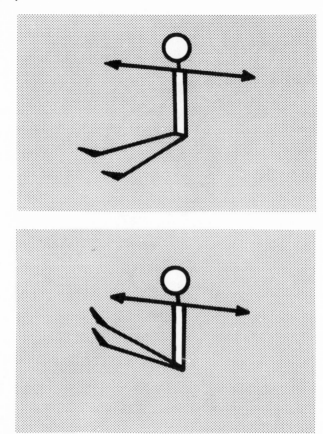

tate her; don't invent a new excuse each day for postponing the self-imposed exercise program. Pay special attention to your weak points, and don't mind sweating a little—there is nothing wrong with sweating!

1) AWAY WITH THE BELLY!

Sit erect on the floor with legs stretched out in front of you, knees straight. Arms are extended sideways at shoulder level. Now raise your legs slightly. Don't brace yourself with your hands—the arms have to stay stretched out sideways during the entire exercise. Then alternately shift one leg over the

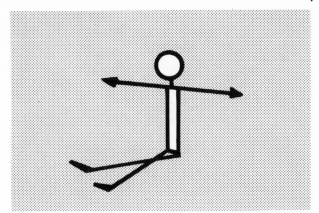

other. For a variation, whip the legs up and down. Now, repeat the process in a livelier tempo, if you please.

2) HAPPILY HIPLESS!

Lying relaxed on your back, stretch the arms sideways at shoulder level, with your palms on the floor. Be sure to keep your shoulders on the floor throughout this exercise. Keeping the stretched legs together, raise them to form a right angle with your trunk. From this position, slowly lower the legs sideways to the floor toward the outstretched left arm, return legs to center position, and slowly lower them toward the right arm.

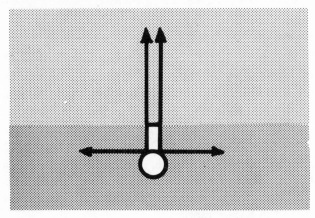

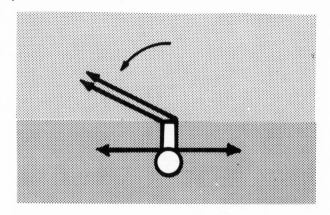

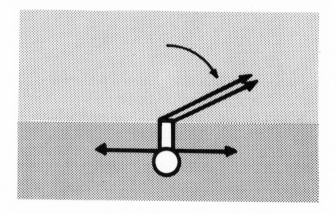

3) FIRMING UP THE FANNY

You sit on the floor, legs stretched out in front, knees straight, arms slightly back with palms on floor, fingertips pointing forward. Raise the stretched left leg to form a right angle with your body and swing it to the left onto the floor. Raise the leg again to a right angle and swing across the body toward the floor on the right. Follow through with the hip all the way, and you will have swung the left leg over the right one. Repeat with the other leg. Don't shift your hands, and don't rest comfortably on your elbows; they may only be bent slightly along with the body's motion.

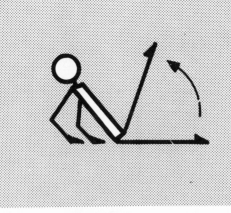

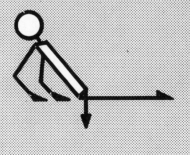

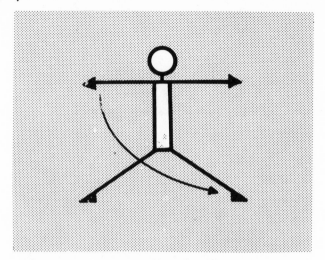

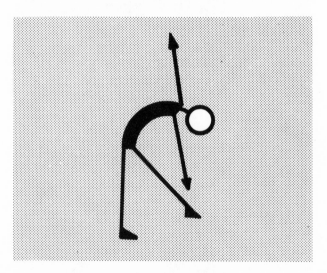

4) A WAISTLINE FIT TO BE SHOWN OFF

For this exercise stand erect, legs slightly apart, arms stretched sideways at shoulder level. Now reach with your right hand for your left toes, while your left arm points back-

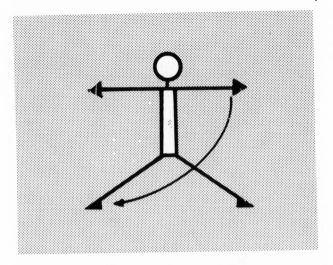

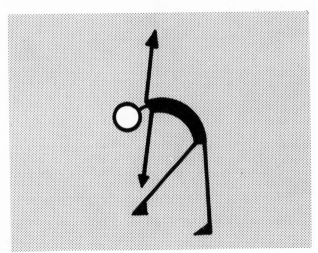

ward. Your head is turned toward your raised left arm and hand. Return to your starting position and carry out the same exercise, but with your left hand reaching toward the right toes. The knees should not be bent. Perform this exercise at a fast clip.

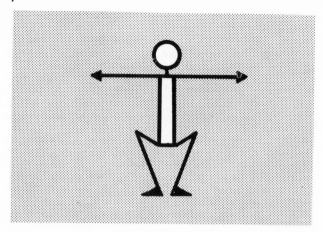

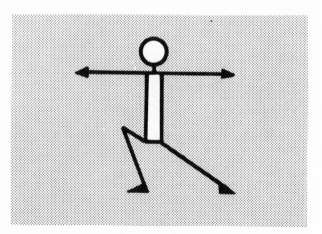

5) THE ROAD TO SHAPELY THIGHS

For this exercise, bend the knees slightly, the arms stretched sideways at chest level. Now take a small jump, swinging the left leg back and stretching it. The right leg stays in the slightly bent position. Now reverse the position of the legs with another jump: You bring the left leg stretched out in back to the front, into the bent posture, and swing the right leg back into the stretched position. The exercise is similar to the lunge in fencing.

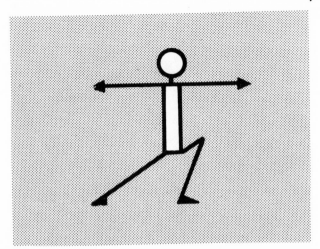

6) FOR A BEAUTIFUL, FIRM BREAST

You sit erect on a stool. Palms are pressed together, finger-tips pointing toward the breast; elbows are raised to shoulder level. Now increase the pressure of the hands against each other while curving breast and breastbone upward. After five seconds, relax the pressure and take a brief rest before repeating the exercise several more times. Another good exercise for keeping the breast in shape is breast-stroke swimming.

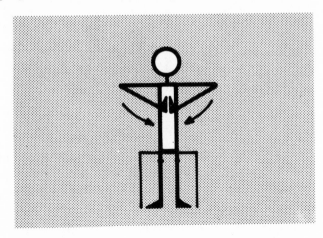

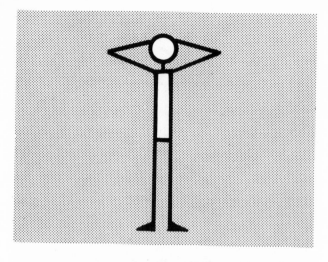

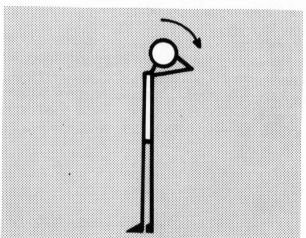

7) DEFENSE AGAINST THE DOUBLE CHIN

Stand erect, hands folded behind your head. As you bend the head backward, exert counterpressure with your hands. Hold this position for a few seconds, relax briefly, and repeat the exercise.

Now, continue the exercise in the opposite direction: Place

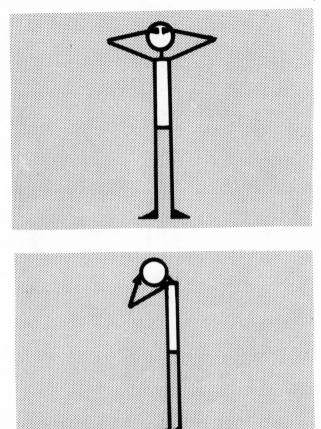

your hands flat on your forehead or make fists. While you are lowering your head until your chin touches your breast, exert a definite counterpressure on your forehead with your hands. Remain in this position for a few seconds, briefly relax, and repeat a few times.

8) TO CONCLUDE: ENDING EXERCISES

Always finish your program with an easy relaxation exercise: Standing upright with your legs together and your arms raised, inhale deeply. Then exhale, allowing the upper part of

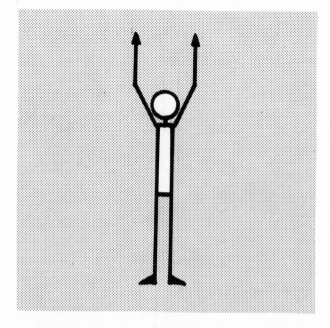

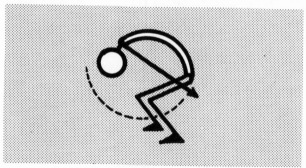

your body to fall forward while relaxing your shoulders and arms. Bend your knees slightly and swing your arms back and forth until they are totally relaxed.

We are not after records with our exercises; you should only work up some sweat. Perhaps you can find a way to perform your exercises together with your children, friends, or acquaintances; such a group effort often improves your performance and makes it easier to exercise regularly. You may want to turn on the radio or play your favorite record—that will surely get you into the swing.

Don't lose heart if an exercise doesn't succeed on the first try; the aim is not to present a pretty picture, but only to carry out the exercise effectively. If you regularly perform the indicated exercises—you may vary them according to inclination and mood—you will soon feel their effect. In a short time, you will notice that your skin and muscles have gained tone and elasticity. You can additionally improve the condition of your skin and body tissues by hot and cold showers, and by massage with a brush.

TOO INDOLENT FOR A FEW SECONDS OF ACUPRESSURE? HOW WOULD YOU LIKE TO TRY WIRE, KNIFE, AND ELECTRICITY?

I am firmly convinced that my combination of acupressure plus diet, backed up by suitable exercise is, in fact, the only effective, lasting method to overcome compulsive eating and obesity, both for the individual and for wider application, since we are faced here with an extremely costly threat to public health. I am further convinced that acupressure makes reducing as easy and painless as is possible.

Yet, I have no illusions that there are not certain individuals who consider even that too much, who want to make it still easier for themselves. For these people I want to list a few other possibilities that still remain:

1) SEW UP THE MOUTH

In Adelaide, Australia, one dental surgeon uses the following method to fight obesity: In the area of the upper and lower canines he attaches loops which he then wires together in such a way that the mouth can be opened only to a narrow slit just sufficient to admit liquid food, nothing else. The patients are fed an 800-calorie mixture of milk, tomato juice, and fruit

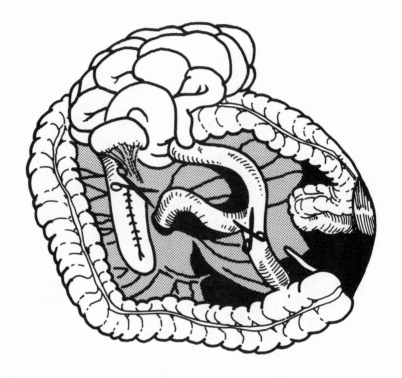

juice, supplemented by multivitamins. They do, indeed, lose weight fast. They also lose the capacity to laugh since they now cannot open the mouth wide enough.

2) OUT WITH THE INTESTINES

One can attack the problem of excessive fat accumulation also from the other end: not less food, but less digestion. This is accomplished by shortening the digestive tract—that is, the intestines—by a surgical procedure that puts out of commission a longish section of healthy small intestine. It is a procedure for the fearless who are willing to undergo major surgery, with all

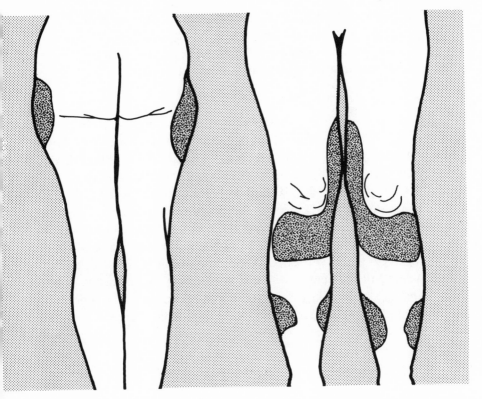

its attendant risks, for the sake of reducing the effects of their gluttony!

3) GET SLIM IN YOUR SLEEP

That is tops for the really lazy: One lies in bed or lounges in a chair watching television, with a few "muscle stimulators" attached to the unwanted fatty deposits, and has within easy reach an "electric stimulator"—and all that for less than five hundred dollars. If one presses a little button, the muscles are supposedly stimulated, and the fat disappears as if by magic. Wouldn't that be great!

The only problem is that the muscles don't have the slightest intention of working off the fat because of some weak electrical goading. They do that only when they have to expend energy. So, the electro-reducing is merely a beautiful dream from which the dreamer wakes up just as fat as before.

4) SIMPLY CUT IT OFF

That is surely the most straightforward approach: Why try to get at the fat via involved detours like diet, shortening of the intestines, or wiring up the jaws, when one can attack it directly? Simply cut off the bothersome fat bulges—that's it! Although you may find it hard to believe, this is feasible and is being done. The skin over the pillow of fat is cut open and folded out, the fat is removed, the skin is turned back—usually somewhat cropped, because by now it is too wide—and stitched together again. Finished. Once the wound, with luck, has healed, the patient's compulsion to eat is by no means gone, and the body takes its revenge for the rude interference: It rebuilds fatty tissue on the exact spot from where it was removed.

APPENDIX/ THE SCIENTIFIC BASIS OF ACUPRESSURE

FOR MANY READERS ALL THAT MATTERS IS THAT ACUPRESSURE works. Why it works does not interest them. They want to lose weight, and do not want to be bored by graphs of neurotransmitters and their effects. On the other hand, there are readers interested in science, and my medical colleagues who might like to know about the scientific basis of acupressure. To satisfy both these groups, I present some important scientific fundamentals of acupressure in this Appendix.

CHANGE IN NEUROTRANSMITTERS

Two million operations were performed in the People's Republic of China (up to the end of 1976) under acupuncture anesthesia, and not a single death due to this type of anesthesia was registered. This created a worldwide stir, since under traditional chemical anesthesia the same number of operations could have been expected to result in 100 fatalities. By now, about 3,000 operations under acupuncture anesthesia have been performed in Germany, and there, too, this procedure has proved beneficial because it is devoid of danger for the patient. Less well known is the fact that operations have also been successfully performed in China under acupressure anesthesia, including operations in the region of the abdomen and of the head, and gynecological surgery.

For several years now, scientists have been investigating the successful release of reflexes, through acupuncture and acupressure, for the suppression of pain or compulsion. First it was proven, in numerous animal experiments, that acupuncture and acupressure have nothing to do with hypnosis or autosuggestion. As I noted earlier, several Caesarean sections have been done on beef cattle by a veterinarian under acupuncture anesthesia. By now, several acupuncture animal hospitals have been established in the United States, where acupressure and acupuncture are used mainly in the treatment of valuable racehorses.

One of the main research centers for scientific animal experiments in acupuncture and acupressure in China is the

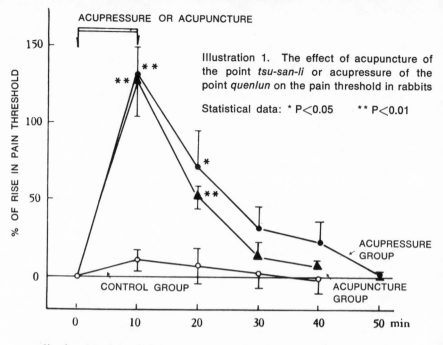

ACUPRESSURE OR ACUPUNCTURE

Illustration 1. The effect of acupuncture of the point *tsu-san-li* or acupressure of the point *quenlun* on the pain threshold in rabbits

Statistical data: * P<0.05   ** P<0.01

medical school in Peking. During my study trips to China in 1974 and 1975, I was able to observe Dr. Han Chi-sheng demonstrate on rabbits the possibility of releasing reflexes in the brain by means of acupressure, and the subsequent changes in the neurotransmitters. These substances not only influence pain sensitivity but also, and especially, eating compulsion.

Dr. Sebastian P. Grossman of the University of Chicago recently reported on pertinent studies: *By targeted interference with a certain neurotransmitter (serotonin) in the brain, hyperphagia (overeating) could be experimentally induced in animals.* It is exactly this neurotransmitter that is being influenced by acupressure. What particular effect is to be achieved, whether it is suppression of pain or of eating compulsion, depends solely on the choice of the point to be stimulated. This means that the overeater's acupressure influences only compulsive eating, and not the pain threshold; other acupressure points influence only the sensitivity to pain. By analogy, in both cases the *same thing* must be happening in the brain, but in different brain centers: *The working of the neurotransmitters is being altered.*

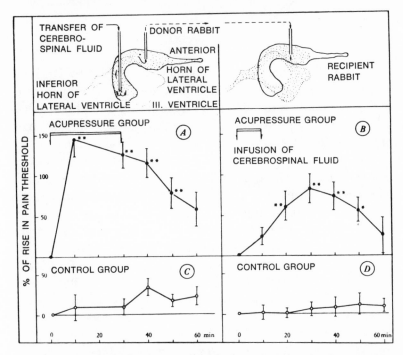

Illustration 2. Effect of acupressure in experiment with transfusion of cerebrospinal fluid   Statistical data: * P<0.05   ** P<0.01

This is proven by the example of the pain-suppressing points: at the medical school in Peking, we were shown (Illustration 1) how the pain threshold rises by 128 percent after acupuncture of the point *tsu-san-li* (shown by curve with triangles), and further, how the pain threshold rises in similar fashion, namely by 133 percent (shown by dotted curve) after acupressure of the point *quenlun,* with a massage frequency of two movements per second. As in all scientific experiments, a control group was included (shown by curve with small circles) to measure the difference in pain threshold. Each animal group comprised ten rabbits. The method and measuring arrangements were the following: a strong heat-beam was aimed at the sensitive nostrils of a blindfolded rabbit. The scientist clocked the time it took for the animal to give a clear sign of pain by turning its head sideways, away from the hot beam (Illustration 2).

Even more impressive was another experiment by Dr. Han, where a group of sixteen rabbits was used. Dr. Han took cerebrospinal fluid from one rabbit (the donor rabbit) that had undergone acupressure with subsequent rise in the pain threshold, and transferred the fluid into a brain ventricle of a second rabbit (the recipient). This second rabbit also showed the very definite rise in pain threshold of 82 percent, while this effect was missing in a control group that had not undergone acupressure (Illustration 3). *This was positive proof that correctly applied acupressure changes neurotransmitters in the brain.* The internationally recognized Viennese professor Dr. Birkmayer, chief of the Ludwig Boltzmann Institute for Neurochemistry, also investigated human neurotransmitters after acupuncture and his findings confirmed those of the Chinese scientists. Related research is presently being done at the University of Munich. Dr. Han further reported on the scientific research going on at the Peking medical school: Electrophysiological investigation of experimental animals has shown that strong pressure on muscles and tendons clearly impedes the neural discharge in the nonspecific nuclei of the thalamus in rats and rabbits, as well as in the reticular system (a netlike brain tissue) of the brain stem in guinea pigs.

It would go beyond the scope of this book to cite the other scientific experiments with animals under acupressure. The interested reader may turn to the Chinese publication *Scientia sinica* (English edition), Vol. 17, No. 1, February 1974, which can be ordered from: Guozi Shudian, China Publications Center, P.O. Box 399, Peking, People's Republic of China.

For a discussion of the compulsive eating center, see Dr. Sebastian P. Grossman, "The Neuroanatomy of Eating and Drinking Behavior," published in *Hospital Practice,* May 1977.

INDEX

Acupressure
  combined with diet, importance of, 25
  dangers from excessive or neurotic use of, 47
  degree of the pressure, 31
  direction of the massage, 31
  general data on, 26–29
  history of, 26
  as a method for everyone, 45–46
  operations performed under, 153–156
  oral reflexes and, 36
  pincer, 34–36
  point of, 32–34
    locating, 30–31
  reactions of patients to, 121–127
  self-administration of, 28–29
  sexual activity and, 36
  stickers, 37
Acupuncture, 26–29, 32
  operations performed under, 153–154
  points of, 27, 28
  workings of, 27–28
Addiction
  alcoholism, 25
  eating as, 21–23, 25
  narcotics, 25
  smoking, 25
Alcoholic beverages
  the banquet and, 20
  diets and, 65, 92
  exercise and, 133
  overweight and, 12, 15, 20
Alcoholism, 25
Animals, domesticated, 22–23
Antidepressants, 42
Appetite, 21, 22, 25
Attractiveness, overweight and, 11
Autonomic nervous system, 21, 27

Banquets, 20
Between-meal snacks, 49, 64
Beverages
  diets and, 48, 64–65, 92
  See also Alcoholic beverages

Bicycle riding, 132
Birkmayer, Dr., 156
Blood-pressure checks, 62–63
Bowel functions, 61
Brain, the, 21–23, 28
  depression and, 39
Breast feeding, 18–19
Breasts, exercises for, 145
Build and Blood Pressure Study, 15
Buttocks, exercise for, 140

Calcium, 57
Calories
  average consumption, 18
  average requirements, 18
  the banquet and, 20
Carbohydrates, 56, 61
  metabolism of, 11
Cardiac infarction, 11, 12
Children
  overfed, 16, 23, 45
  overweight, 23
China, People's Republic of, 153–156
Cholesterol, 11
Cirrhosis of the liver, 12
Compulsive eaters, test for determining, 31–32
Compulsive eating, 21–23, 25
  conditioning against, 29–30
Conditioned reflexes, 29
  for compulsive eating, 29–30
Crash diets, 51–55

Dancing, 133
Depression, 38–42
  the brain and, 39
  restlessness during, 41–42
Diabetes, 58
Diets, 23–25, 47–120
  acupressure combined with, importance of, 25
  between-meal snacks, 49, 64
  beverages and, 48, 64–65, 92
  alcoholic, 65, 92

Diets (*cont.*)
  blood-pressure checks and, 62–63
  the body needs, 55–58
    carbohydrates, 56
    fats, 56–57
    fillers, 57–58
    minerals, 57
    proteins, 55
    vitamins, 57
  bowel functions, 61
  choosing, 58
  crash, 51–55
  creating a feeling of fullness, 48–49
  drinking before meals, 48
  eating slowly, 49
  ground rules for, 48–51
  leftovers, attitude toward, 50–51
  shopping for food, 49–50
  small helpings, 49
  variety in foods, 66
  weight-maintenance, 93–120
  250-300 calorie, 58–65
  800-calorie, 65–91
  1300-calorie, 93–120
Double chin, exercise for, 146–147
Drugs, 12
  addiction to, 25
  antidepressants, 42

Eating habits, 15–23
  average caloric consumption, 18
  average caloric requirements, 18
  banquets, 20
  compulsive eaters, test for determining, 31–32
  compulsive eating, 21–23, 25
    conditioning against, 29–30
  eating as an addiction, 21–23, 25
  grievance fat, 19
  hard labor and, 17–18
  inherited from the past, 16–18
  nervous eating, 19
  the pleasure function, 16–17
  stress and, 18–20, 42–44
  stretch receptors and, 37–38
  substitute gratification, 19
800-calorie diet, 65–91
Endogenous depressions, 39
Energy
  average requirements, 18
  the banquet and, 20
  control mechanism for, 21–23
  storing reserves of, 16
  stress and, 19–20
Exercise, 127–149
  advisable limit of, 130
  alcoholic beverages and, 133
  bicycle riding, 132
  dancing, 133
  fat and, 128–129
  hiking, 130–131
  overweight and, 23
  pulse rate during, 130
  running, 130–131
  swimming, 131–132

Exercises, 133–149
  aimed at critical points, 137–147
  ending, 147–149
  jumping jack, 135
  knee bends, 135–136
  rope jumping, 134–135
  running in place, 134
Exogenous depressions, 39

Fasting, 51–52
Fat(s), 56–57
  average consumption of, 18
  the banquet and, 20
  exercise and, 128–129
  grievance, 19
  hard labor and, 17–18
  hibernation and, 22
  metabolism of, 11
  storing, 16
Fawcett-Majors, Farrah, 137–138
Fillers, 48–49, 57–58
Francisco, Dr. Jerry, 12
Fruit, 61–62, 66
Frustrations, 44

Gallbladder cramps, 12
Gallstones, overweight and, 12
German Academy for Auricular Medicine, 29
German Internists, Congress of, 51
Goethe, Johann Wolfgang von, 17
Gout, 58
Gratification, substitute, 19
Grievance fat, 19
Grossman, Dr. Sebastian P., 154, 156

Han Chi-sheng, Dr., 154–156
Hard labor, 17–18
Headaches, 12
Heart, the, overweight and, 11, 12
Hibernation, fat and, 22
High blood pressure, overweight and, 11–12
Hiking, 130–131
Hips, exercise for, 139
Hospital Practice, 156
Hunger, 21–22
Hypothalamus, the, 21–22

Ideal weight, 13–15
  bone structure and, 14
  defined, 13
  men, 14
  women, 15

Jumping jack, 135

Kennedy, Donald, 60
Kidney stones, 58
Kissing, 36
Knee bends, 135–136

Labor, hard, 17–18
Leftovers, attitudes toward, 23, 50–51
Life expectancy, overweight and, 12
Liver, the, cirrhosis of, 12

Ludwig Boltzmann Institute for Neurochemistry, 156

Massaging, direction of, 31
Men
  average energy requirement, 18
  ideal weight, 14
  opinions of, statistics on, 13
Menus
  250-300 calorie diet, 58–65
  800-calorie diet, 65–91
  1300-calorie diet, 93–120
Metabolism
  carbohydrates, 11
  fats, 11
Metropolitan Life Insurance Company, 14–15
Midbrain, the, 21, 25, 28
Minerals, 57, 60
Multivitamin tablets, 61–62

Narcotic addiction, 25
National Center for Health Statistics, 13
Nervous eating, 19
Nervous system, 21, 27
"Neuroanatomy of Eating and Drinking Behavior, The" (Grossman), 156
Neurotransmitters, 154–156
Nutrition, utilizing internal, 16

Obesity, see Overweight
Operations
  for overweight, 149–152
  performed under acupressure, 153–156
  performed under acupuncture, 153–154
Oral reflexes, acupressure and, 36
Overeating, see Eating habits
Overfed children, 16, 23, 45
Overweight
  alcoholic beverages and, 12, 15, 20
  attractiveness and, 11
  carbohydrate metabolism and, 11
  children, 23
  dangers of, 11–13
  eating habits and, 15–23
    average caloric consumption, 18
    average caloric requirements, 18
    banquets, 20
    compulsive eaters, test for determining, 31–32
    compulsive eating, 21–23, 25
    conditioning against compulsive eating, 29–30
    eating as an addiction, 21–23, 25
    grievance fat, 19
    hard labor and, 17–18
    inherited from the past, 16–18
    nervous eating, 19
    the pleasure function, 16–17
    stress and, 18–20, 42–44
    stretch receptors and, 37–38
    substitute gratification, 19
  exercise and, 23
  fat metabolism and, 11
  gallstones and, 12

the heart and, 11, 12
high blood pressure and, 11–12
life expectancy and, 12
the liver and, 12
operations for, 149–152
statistics on, 13

Parasympathetic nervous system, 27
Pavlov, Ivan Petrovich, 29
Pincer acupressure, 34–36
Pleasure
  eating and, 16–17
  reproduction and, 17
Potassium, 57, 60, 61
Presley, Elvis, 12
Pressure, degree of, 31
Protein(s), 55
  concentrates, 60
  raw vegetables and, 60–61
Pulse rate during exercise, 130

Reflexes, conditioned, 29
  for compulsive eating, 29–30
Reproduction, pleasure in the process of, 17
Restlessness during depression, 41–42
Rope jumping, 134–135
Running, 130–131
Running in place, 134

Satiety, 21, 22
Scientia sinica, 156
Seitz, Helmut, 52–54
Sexual activity
  acupressure and, 36
  pleasure in, 17
Sleep, disturbance of, 12
Smoking, addiction to, 25
Society of Actuaries, 15
Starvation, 16, 25
Stickers, 37
Stomach exercises, 138–139
Stress, 18–20, 42–44
  energy and, 19–20
Stress reaction, 19–20
Stretch receptors, 37–38
Substitute gratification, 19
Süddeutsche Zeitung, 52–54
Swimming, 131–132
Sympathetic nervous system, 27

Thighs, exercise for, 144
1300-calorie diet, 93–120
250-300 calorie diet, 58–65

Underweight, statistics on, 13
U. S. Food and Drug Administration, 60

Vegetables, raw, 48–49, 58, 66
  proteins and, 60–61
Vitamins, 57, 60
  multivitamin tablets, 61–62

Waistline, exercise for, 142–143
Weight-maintenance diet, 93–120

Women
  average energy requirement, 18
  cooking methods of, 17
  ideal weight, 15
  opinions of, statistics on, 13

Yin-Yang principle, 27
Yogurt, 61, 62

Zehn-shi, 26